Evidence-based Clinical Chinese Medicine

Volume 23
Episodic Migraine

Evidence-based Clinical Chinese Medicine

Print ISSN: 2529-7562
Online ISSN: 2529-7554

Series Co Editors-in-Chief

Charlie Changli Xue *(RMIT University, Australia)*
Chuanjian Lu *(Guangdong Provincial Hospital of Chinese Medicine, China)*

Published

More information on this series can also be found at https://www.worldscientific.com/series/ebccm

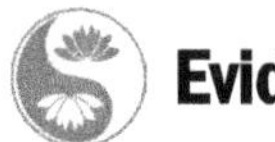

Evidence-based Clinical Chinese Medicine

Co Editors-in-Chief

Charlie Changli Xue
RMIT University, Australia

Chuanjian Lu
Guangdong Provincial Hospital of Chinese Medicine, China

Volume 23
Episodic Migraine

Lead Authors

Claire Shuiqing Zhang
RMIT University, Australia

Shaohua Lyu
Guangdong Provincial Hospital of Chinese Medicine, China

World Scientific

NEW JERSEY · LONDON · SINGAPORE · BEIJING · SHANGHAI · HONG KONG · TAIPEI · CHENNAI · TOKYO

Published by

World Scientific Publishing Co. Pte. Ltd.

5 Toh Tuck Link, Singapore 596224

USA office: 27 Warren Street, Suite 401-402, Hackensack, NJ 07601

UK office: 57 Shelton Street, Covent Garden, London WC2H 9HE

Library of Congress Cataloging-in-Publication Data
Names: Xue, Charlie Changli, author. | Lu, Chuan-jian, 1964–   author.
Title: Evidence-based clinical Chinese medicine / Charlie Changli Xue, Chuanjian Lu.
Description: New Jersey : World Scientific, 2016. | Includes bibliographical references and index.
Identifiers: LCCN 2015030389| ISBN 9789814723084 (v. 1 : hardcover : alk. paper) |
   ISBN 9789814723091 (v. 1 : paperback : alk. paper) |
   ISBN 9789814723121 (v. 2 : hardcover : alk. paper) |
   ISBN 9789814723138 (v. 2 : paperback : alk. paper) |
   ISBN 9789814759045 (v. 3 : hardcover : alk. paper) |
   ISBN 9789814759052 (v. 3 : paperback : alk. paper)
Subjects: | MESH: Medicine, Chinese Traditional--methods. | Clinical Medicine--methods. |
   Evidence-Based Medicine--methods. | Psoriasis. | Pulmonary Disease, Chronic Obstructive.
Classification: LCC RC81 | NLM WB 55.C4 | DDC 616--dc23
LC record available at http://lccn.loc.gov/2015030389

Volume 23: Episodic Migraine
ISBN 978-981-123-393-7 (hardcover)
ISBN 978-981-123-546-7 (paperback)
ISBN 978-981-123-394-4 (ebook for institutions)
ISBN 978-981-123-395-1 (ebook for individuals)

British Library Cataloguing-in-Publication Data
A catalogue record for this book is available from the British Library.

For any available supplementary material, please visit
https://www.worldscientific.com/worldscibooks/10.1142/12197#t=suppl

Disclaimer

The information in this book is based on systematic analyses of the best available evidence for Chinese medicine interventions both historical and contemporary. Every effort has been made to ensure accuracy and completeness of the data herein. This book is intended for clinicians, researchers and educators. The practice of evidence-based medicine consists of consideration of the best available evidence, practitioners' clinical experience and judgment, and patients' preference. Not all interventions are acceptable in all countries. It is important to note that some of the substances mentioned in this book may no longer be in use, may be toxic, or may be prohibited or restricted under the provisions of the Convention on International Trade in Endangered Species of Wild Fauna and Flora (CITES). Practitioners, researchers and educators are advised to comply with the relevant regulations in their country and with the restrictions on the trade in species included in CITES appendices I, II and III. This book is not intended as a guide for self-medication. Patients should seek professional advice from qualified Chinese medicine practitioners.

Foreword

Since the late 20th century, Chinese medicine, including acupuncture and herbal medicine, has been increasingly used throughout the world. The parallel development and spread of evidence-based medicine have provided challenges and opportunities for Chinese medicine. The opportunities have been evidence-based medicine's emphasis on the effective use of the best available clinical evidence, incorporating the clinicians' clinical experience, subject to patients' preference. Such practices have a patient focus which reflects the historical nature of Chinese medicine practice. However, the challenges are also significant due to the fact that, despite the long-term development and very rich literature accumulated over 2,000 years, there is an overall lack of high-level clinical evidence for many of the interventions used in Chinese medicine.

To address this knowledge gap, we need to generate clinical evidence through high-quality clinical studies and to evaluate evidence to enable effective use of such available evidence to promote evidence-based Chinese medicine practice.

Modern Chinese medicine is rooted in its classical literature and the legacies of ancient doctors, grounded in the practice of expert clinicians and increasingly informed by clinical and experimental research efforts. In recognition of the unique features of Chinese medicine, for each of the conditions in this series a 'whole-evidence' approach is used to provide a synthesis of different types and levels of evidence to enable practitioners to make clinical decisions informed by the current best evidence.

There are four main components of this 'whole-evidence' approach. In the first component, we present the current approaches to the diagnosis, differentiation and treatment of each condition based on expert consensus in published textbooks and clinical guidelines. This provides an overview of how the condition is currently managed. The second component provides an analysis of the condition in historical context based on systematic searches of the *Zhong Hua Yi Dian* 中华医典 which includes the full texts of more than 1,000 classical medical books. These analyses provide objective views on how the condition has been treated over two millennia, reveal continuities and discontinuities between traditional and modern practice, and suggest avenues for future research.

The third component is the assessment of evidence derived from modern clinical studies of Chinese medicine interventions. The methods established by the *Cochrane Collaboration* are used as the basis for conducting systematic reviews and undertaking meta-analyses of outcome data for randomised controlled trials (RCTs). In addition, the clinical relevance of meta-analysis data is enhanced by examining the herbal formulas, individual herbs and acupuncture treatments that were assessed in the RCTs and the evidence base is broadened by the inclusion of data from controlled clinical trials and non-controlled studies. The fourth component is to determine how the herbal medicine interventions may achieve the effects indicated by the clinical trials. Thus for each of the most frequently used herbs we provide reviews of their effects in pre-clinical models and their likely mechanisms of action.

For each condition, this 'whole-evidence' approach links clinical expertise, historical precedent, clinical research data and experimental research to provide the reader with assessments of the current state of the evidence for the efficacy, effectiveness and safety of Chinese medicine interventions using herbal medicines, acupuncture and moxibustion and other health care practices such as *tuina* 推拿 therapy.

Since these books are available in Chinese and English, they can benefit patients, practitioners and educators internationally and enable practitioners to make clinical decisions informed by the current best evidence.

These publications represent a major milestone in the development of Chinese medicine and make a significant contribution to the development of evidence-based Chinese medicine globally.

Co-Editors-in-Chief

Distinguished Professor Charlie Changli Xue,
RMIT University, Australia

Professor Chuanjian Lu, Guangdong Provincial Hospital of
Chinese Medicine, China

Purpose of the Book

This book is intended for clinicians, researchers and educators. It can be used to inform tertiary education and clinical practice by providing systematic, multi-dimensional assessments of the best available evidence for using Chinese medicine to manage each common clinical condition.

How to Use This Book

Some Definitions

A glossary is included, containing terms and definitions which frequently appear in the book. It also describes the definitions of statistical tests, methodological terms, evaluation tools and interventions. For example, in this book, integrative medicine refers to the combined use of a Chinese medicine treatment with conventional medical management, and combination therapies refer to two or more Chinese medicines from different therapy groups (Chinese herbal medicine, acupuncture or other Chinese medicine therapies) administered together. Terminology used throughout the book is based on the World Health Organization's *Standard Terminologies on Traditional Medicine in the Western Pacific Region* (2007) where possible or from the cited reference.

Data Analysis and Interpretation of Results

In order to synthesise the clinical evidence, a range of statistical analysis approaches is used. In general, the effect size for dichotomous data is reported as a risk ratio (RR) with 95% confidence interval (CI), and for continuous data, they are reported as mean difference (MD) with 95% CI. Statistically significant effects are indicated with an asterisk*. Readers should note that statistical significance does not necessarily correspond with a clinically important effect. Interpretation of results should take into consideration the clinical significance, quality of studies (expressed as high, low or unclear risk of bias in this book) and heterogeneity amongst the studies. Tests for heterogeneity are conducted using the I^2 statistic. An I^2 score greater than 50% may indicate substantial heterogeneity.

Use of Evidence in Practice

The Grading of Recommendations Assessment, Development and Evaluation (GRADE) approach was used to summarise the results and certainty of the evidence for critical and important comparisons and outcomes. Due to the diverse nature of Chinese medicine practice, treatment recommendations are not included with the summary-of-findings tables. Therefore, readers will need to interpret the evidence with reference to the local practice environment.

Limitations

Readers should note some of the methodological limitations of the classical literature and the clinical evidence.

- Search terms used to search the *Zhong Hua Yi Dian* 中华医典 database may not include all terms that have been used for the condition, which may alter the findings.
- Chinese language has changed over time. Citations have been interpreted for analysis, and such interpretations may be subject to disagreement.
- Chinese medicine theory has evolved over time. As such, concepts described in classical Chinese medical literature may no longer be found in contemporary works.

- Symptoms described in citations may be common to many conditions, and a judgment was required to determine the likelihood of the citation being related to the condition. This may have introduced some bias due to the subjective nature of the judgment.
- The vast majority of the clinical evidence for Chinese medicine treatments has come from China. The applicability of the findings to other populations and other countries requires further assessment.
- Many studies included participants with varying disease severity. Where possible, subgroup analyses were undertaken to examine the effects in different subpopulations. As this was not always possible, the findings may be limited to the population included, and not to subpopulations.
- The potential risk of bias found in many included studies suggested methodological limitations. The findings for GRADE assessments based on studies of very low to moderate quality evidence should be interpreted accordingly.
- Nine major English- and Chinese-language databases were searched to identify clinical studies, in addition to clinical trial registers. Other studies may exist which were not identified through searches, and which may alter the findings.
- The calculation of frequency of herbal formula use was based on formula names. It is possible that studies evaluated herbal treatments with the same or similar herb ingredients, but which were given different formula names. Due to the complexity of herbal formulas, it was considered not appropriate to make a judgment as to the similarity of formulas for analysis. As such, the frequency of formulas reported in Chapter 5 may be underestimated.
- The most frequently utilised herbs which may have contributed to the treatment effect have been described in Chapter 5. These herbs may provide leads for further exploration. Calculation of the herbs with potential effect is based on frequency of formulas reported in the studies, and does not take into consideration the clinical implications and functions of every herb in a formula.

Authors and Contributors

Co-Editors-in-Chief

Distinguished Prof. Charlie Changli Xue (*RMIT University, Australia*)
Prof. Chuanjian Lu (*Guangdong Provincial Hospital of Chinese Medicine, China*)

Co-Deputy Editors-in-Chief

Assoc. Prof. Anthony Lin Zhang (*RMIT University, Australia*)
Dr. Brian H May (*RMIT University, Australia*)
Prof. Xinfeng Guo (*Guangdong Provincial Hospital of Chinese Medicine, China*)
Prof. Zehuai Wen (*Guangdong Provincial Hospital of Chinese Medicine, China*)

Lead Authors

Dr. Claire Shuiqing Zhang (*RMIT University, Australia*)
Dr. Shaohua Lyu (*Guangdong Provincial Hospital of Chinese Medicine, China*)

Co-Authors

RMIT University (Australia):
Dr. Mary Xinmei Zhang
Assoc. Prof. Anthony Lin Zhang
Distinguished Prof. Charlie Changli Xue

Guangdong Provincial Hospital of Chinese Medicine (China):

Prof. Chuanjian Lu
Prof. Xiaodong Luo
Prof. Xinfeng Guo
Prof. Qiaozhen Su

Members of Advisory Committee and Panel

CO-CHAIRS OF PROJECT PLANNING COMMITTEE

Prof. Peter J Coloe (*RMIT University, Australia*)
Prof. Yubo Lyu (*Guangdong Provincial Hospital of Chinese Medicine, China*)
Prof. Dacan Chen (*Guangdong Provincial Hospital of Chinese Medicine, China*)

CENTRE ADVISORY COMMITTEE (IN ALPHABETICAL ORDER)

Prof. Keji Chen (*The Chinese Academy of Sciences, China*)
Prof. Aiping Lu (*Hong Kong Baptist University, China*)
Prof. Caroline Smith (*University of Western Sydney, Australia*)
Prof. David F Story (*RMIT University, Australia*)

METHODOLOGY EXPERT ADVISORY PANEL (IN ALPHABETICAL ORDER)

Prof. Zhaoxiang Bian (*Hong Kong Baptist University, China*)
Prof. Lixing Lao (*The University of Hong Kong, China*)
The Late Prof. George Lewith (*University of Southampton, United Kingdom*)
Prof. Jianping Liu (*Beijing University of Chinese Medicine, China*)
Prof. Frank Thien (*Monash University, Australia*)
Prof. Jialiang Wang (*Sichuan University, China*)

CONTENT EXPERT ADVISORY PANEL (IN ALPHABETICAL ORDER)

Prof. Bin Li (*Beijing Hospital of Chinese Medicine, Beijing, China*)
Prof. Wei Xie (*Nanfang Hospital, Southern Medical University, Guangdong, China*)
Prof. Jingsong You (*Guangdong Provincial Hospital of Chinese Medicine, Guangdong, China*)
Prof. Fang Zeng (*Chengdu University of Chinese Medicine, Sichuan, China*)

Distinguished Professor
Charlie Changli Xue

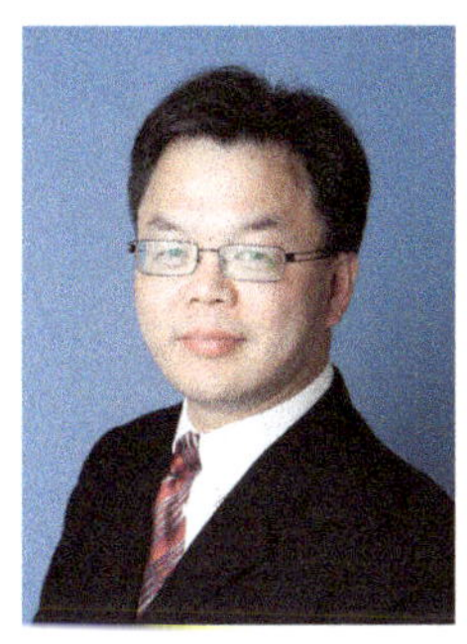

Distinguished Professor Charlie Changli Xue holds a Bachelor of Medicine (majoring in Chinese Medicine) from Guangzhou University of Chinese Medicine, China (1987) and a PhD from RMIT University, Australia (2000). He has been an academic, researcher, regulator and practitioner for almost three decades. Professor Xue has made significant contributions to evidence-based educational development, clinical research, regulatory framework and policy development and provision of high-quality clinical care to the community. Professor Xue is recognised internationally as an expert in evidence-based traditional medicine and integrative health care.

Professor Xue is the Inaugural National Chair of the Chinese Medicine Board of Australia appointed by the Australian Health Workforce Ministerial Council (in 2011), and he was reappointed for a second term in 2014 and a third term in 2017. Since 2007, he has been a Member of the World Health Organization (WHO) Expert Advisory Panel for Traditional and Complementary Medicine, Geneva. Professor Xue is also Honorary Senior Principal Research Fellow at the Guangdong Provincial Academy of Chinese Medical Sciences, China.

At RMIT, Professor Xue is Executive Dean, School of Health and Biomedical Sciences. He is also Director, WHO Collaborating Centre for Traditional Medicine.

Between 1995 and 2010, Professor Xue was Discipline Head of Chinese Medicine at RMIT University. He leads the development of five successful undergraduate and postgraduate degree programmes in Chinese Medicine at RMIT University which is now a global leader in Chinese medicine education and research.

Professor Xue's research has been supported by research grants of over AUD 15 million, including six project grants from the Australian Government's National Health and Medical Research Council (NHMRC) and two Australian Research Council (ARC) grants. He has contributed over 200 publications and has been frequently invited as keynote speaker for numerous national and international conferences. Professor Xue has contributed to over 300 media interviews on issues related to complementary medicine education, research, regulation and practice.

Professor Chuanjian Lu

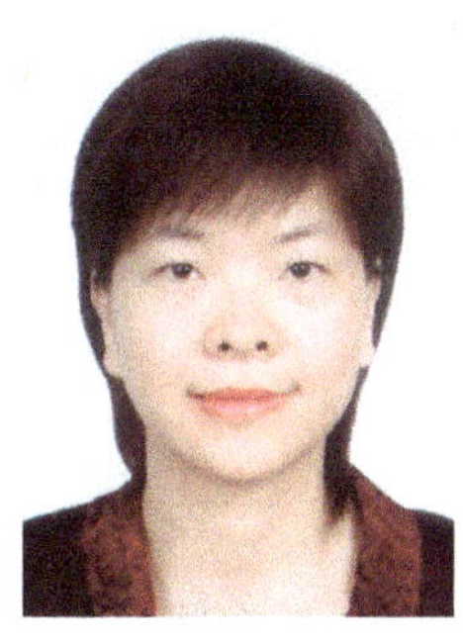

Professor Chuanjian Lu is Vice-president of Guangdong Provincial Hospital of Chinese Medicine (Guangdong Provincial Academy of Chinese Medical Sciences, Second Clinical Medical College of Guangzhou University of Chinese Medicine). She also is Chair of the Guangdong Traditional Chinese Medicine (TCM) Standardisation Technical Committee, and Vice-chair of the Immunity Specialty Committee of the World Federation of Chinese Medicine Societies (WFCMS).

Professor Lu has engaged in scientific research into TCM, clinical practice and teaching for some 25 years. Her research has been devoted to integrating traditional and western medicine. She has edited and published 12 monographs and 120 academic research articles as first author and corresponding author with over 30 articles being included in SCI journals.

She has received widespread recognition for her achievements with awards for Excellent Teacher of South China, National Outstanding Women TCM Doctor and National Outstanding Young Doctor of TCM. She also received the Science and Technology Star of the Association of Chinese Medicine, the National Excellent Science and Technology Workers of China Award and the Five-continent Women's Scientific Award of China Medical Women's Association.

Professor Lu has won the Award of Science and Technology Progress over ten times from Guangdong Provincial Government, China Association of Chinese Medicine and Chinese Hospital Association.

Acknowledgements

The authors and contributors would like to acknowledge the valuable contributions of the following people who assisted with database searches, data extraction, data screening, data assessment, translation of documents, editing and/or administrative tasks: Dr. Jhodie Duncan, Ms. Yanjuan Xu and Ms. Liu Liao.

Contents

Contents

Contents

List of Figures

1

Introduction to Migraine

OVERVIEW

Migraine is the most common severe form of primary headache disorder. Migraine has a significant impact on physical, social and occupational functioning, and it is a significant cause of work absence and disability. This chapter reviews the definition, epidemiology, classification, diagnosis, prognosis and clinical management of migraine.

Definition of Migraine

Migraine is a common disabling primary headache disorder with recurrent episodes of headache attacks lasting from four to 72 hours.[1] Migraine headaches often occur over many years or over an individual's lifetime. The main characteristics of migraine headaches are unilateral location, pulsating quality, moderate or severe intensity, aggravation by routine physical activity and association with nausea, photophobia or phonophobia, or any combination of all these three.[1]

Based on the symptoms, migraine can be divided into major subtypes: migraine without aura and migraine with aura.[1] Most people who have migraine with aura also have attacks of migraine without aura.[1,2]

- Migraine without aura is a clinical syndrome characterised by headache with specific features and associated symptoms.[1]
- Migraine with aura is defined as a 'recurrent disorder manifesting in attacks of reversible focal neurological symptoms that usually develop gradually over five to 20 minutes and last for less than 60 minutes'.[1]

Based on the frequency and duration of headaches, migraine is classified as episodic migraine and chronic migraine:

- Episodic migraine occurs on less than 15 days per month and can be further subdivided into low frequency (1–9 days per month) and high frequency (10–14 days per month).[1]
- Chronic migraine is defined as headache occurring on 15 or more days per month for more than three months, which has the feature of migraine headache on at least eight days per month.[1]

As stated in the International Classification of Headache Disorders, third edition beta version (ICHD-3 beta), chronic migraine is singled out from episodic migraine because it is impossible to distinguish individual episodes of headache in patients with such frequent or continuous headaches. In fact, the characteristics of the headache may change, not only from day to day, but even within the same day. It is extremely difficult to keep such patients free of medication in order to observe the natural history of the headache. In this situation, attacks with or without aura are both counted, as well as tension-type-like headaches. In fact, the most common cause of symptoms suggestive of chronic migraine is medication overuse. Around 50% of patients apparently with chronic migraine revert to an episodic migraine subtype after drug withdrawal; such patients are in a sense wrongly diagnosed as chronic migraine sufferers. Equally, many patients apparently overusing medication do not improve after drug withdrawal, and the diagnosis of medication-overuse headache may, in a sense, be inappropriate (assuming that chronicity induced by drug overuse is always reversible).[1] Due to the fact that chronic migraine is likely mixed with medication-overuse headache, in this book, we have focused on the treatments of episodic migraine (with, or without, aura).

Clinical Presentation of Migraine

The clinical presentation of migraine headache attacks varies greatly in terms of intensity and patterns of associated symptoms. Photophobia, phonophobia, nausea, vomiting, osmophobia, and movement sensitivity occur in different combinations. Auras, characterised by visual symptoms (spots of light, zigzag lines, or graying out of vision), sensory symptoms (tingling and numbness) or language disturbances, occur in 20–30% of people with migraine.[1] The ICHD includes visual (both binocular and monocular), sensory, language, motor and brainstem symptoms as part of the diagnostic criteria for migraine with aura.[1]

Visual aura is the most common type of aura, affecting more than 90% of patients who have migraine with aura, at least in some attacks.[1] It often presents as a fortification spectrum: a zigzag figure near the point of fixation that may gradually spread right or left and assume a laterally convex shape with an angulated scintillating edge, leaving absolute or variable degrees of relative scotoma in its wake.[1] The next most common aura is sensory disturbances, in the form of pins and needles moving slowly from the point of origin and affecting a greater or smaller part of one side of the body, face, and/or tongue. Numbness may occur in its wake, but numbness may also be the only symptom.[1] It was reported that the sensory aura ranged from 30% to 54%.[3,4] Less frequent are speech disturbances, usually aphasic but often hard to categorise. When the speech disturbances also includes motor weakness, such disorder should be coded as hemiplegic migraine or one of its subforms.[1] Speech disturbances have been reported to occur in up to 31% of patients.[4,5] Limited data suggest that the prevalence of motor aura ranges from 6% to 10% of migraine with aura patients or 0.01% of the general population.[6–9] Clinic-based studies have suggested that the prevalence of basilar-type migraine (prior term for brainstem aura in ICHD-I criteria) ranges from 10% in patients with migraine and typical aura, to 75% in patients with familial and sporadic hemiplegic migraine.[10–12]

Patients who suffer from migraine attacks without aura also can have episodes of migraine aura only but without headache.[6,13] The aura typically precedes the headache, but can occur during and even after the headache.[7,14,15] If the headache precedes the aura, it is typically of the tension type.[16] There are also some individuals who experience recurrent auras throughout their lives without ever having a headache.[7,17]

Migraine can present with other types of neurological symptoms. Dizziness or vertigo is fairly common in migraine attacks. At present, there are more data supporting a cortical neuroanatomical basis for migraine-related dizziness.[18–20] Rarely, migraine can present in association with auditory, olfactory and gustatory hallucinations.[21–24] However, given the infrequency of these events, other causes should be investigated as both seizures and stroke have been associated with cortical spreading depression and migrainous headaches.[25–29]

Epidemiology

Migraine is the most common severe form of primary headache with a global prevalence of around one in seven people.[30] The Global Burden of Diseases, Injuries, and Risk Factors Study 2017 (GBD 2017) published results of a global, regional and national epidemiological research on 195 countries, indicating that the prevalence of migraine in 2017 was more than 1,331 million, with approximately 113 million incidences globally.[31]

In fact, migraine is often underdiagnosed, misdiagnosed (e.g. as sinusitis) and undertreated in both primary and secondary care.[32] In a multi-centre primary care-based study, more than 90% of patients presenting to primary care with headache had migraine.[33]

Migraine is more prevalent in females.[34] This is considered to be due to changes in hormone levels during the menstrual cycle, which can be more pronounced at puberty and perimenopause. Before puberty migraine frequency is the same in boys and girls.[35] Following menopause migraine often improves.[35,36] In addition, migraine is more prevalent in those with lower socioeconomic status.[37] Among migraine patients, around 15% to 30% have aura (transient focal neurological symptoms) before or during their headaches.[38] Being consistent with the prevalence of migraine by gender, migraine with aura is more common in women than men.[39] It has been pointed out that, the first incidence of migraine with aura precedes that of migraine without aura by three to five years.[40] On the other hand, auras accompanied the first migraine headache in 39% of the patients.[14] Over time the aura may not be present with every attack and only 19% of patients who have migraine with aura report aura symptoms with every headache attack.[14]

Burden

Migraine has a significant and debilitating impact on physical, social and occupational functioning. It is a significant cause of work absence and disability.[38] More than half of migraineurs report severe impairment or require bed rest during their headaches.[41] Indeed, a study by the World Health Organisation in 2010 showed that migraine is the third most prevalent medical disorder and the eighth most disabling worldwide.[42] The Global Burden of Diseases, Injuries, and Risk Factors Study 2015 (GBD 2015) ranks migraine as the seventh most common cause of disability worldwide, rising to the third most common cause in the under-50s.[43] The most recent GBD 2017 study reported that migraine caused 47.2 million years lived with disability (YLDs) globally in 2017,[31] with an increase of 34.4% from 1990 to 2017.[31]

Migraine also results in a large cost to society, through associated health care costs and loss of productive time.[44–47] For example, a report published in 2010 showed that the estimated cost of migraine in the United Kingdom was around £3 billion a year in direct and indirect costs, taking into consideration the costs of health care, lost productivity and disability.[48]

In Australia, as reported in 2018, the socioeconomic burden of migraine was estimated using best practice cost-of-illness methodology applying a prevalence approach.[49] This approach involves estimating the number of people with migraine in a base period (2018) and the costs attributable to the condition in that period. The analysis was based on the data collected in a targeted data scan and literature review. The key findings of this report are as follows:

- A total of 4.9 million people (20.55% of the whole population) in Australia suffer from migraine; 71% of migraine sufferers are women and 86% are of working age;

- In total 7.6% of migraine sufferers experience chronic migraine (≥15 migraine days per month);
- The total economic cost of migraine in Australia is $35.7 billion. This consists of:
  - $14.3 billion of health system costs;
  - $16.3 billion of productivity costs;
  - $5.1 billion of other costs;
  - Migraine also imposes significant well-being costs on sufferers.

In China, the prevalence of migraine is reported to be 9.3%, with more female than male sufferers (at 3:1 ratio).[50] It is reported by the Global Burden of Disease Study (2016) that the estimated prevalence of migraine in China is about 133 million people resulting in 5.9 million YLDs in 2016.[32]

Triggers in Episodic Migraine

Episodic migraine is a paroxysmal disorder, and the attacks often occur in clusters lasting days or weeks. Many patients with episodic migraine experience headache attacks which varied greatly month-to-month. In most, these fluctuations are not easily explained by common triggers.[51]

It can be challenging to distinguish between migraine triggers and premonitory symptoms which occur two to 48 hours prior to a migraine. The prevalence of premonitory symptoms in migraine varies from 30% to 80%.[52,53] Common premonitory symptoms which may be confused for triggers include neck pain, light sensitivity and food cravings.[54]

Previous studies have focused on exploring the triggers in episodic migraine.[55,56] The confirmed common triggers are described below.

Dietary

There have been dietary studies that attempt to link specific foods to migraine, but due to the lack of placebo, it is difficult to distinguish between premonitory food cravings and migraine triggers. Also, the foods are more likely to be contributory than the sole cause of a migraine attack.[56] Several studies have explored the relationship between migraine and food allergies and have proposed treating migraine with specific diets such as elimination of certain foods.[57,58] Fasting, caffeine withdrawal, and specific foods or additives may also trigger migraine attacks.[56] In addition, it was found that women with migraine had a significantly lower diet quality as reported in a large questionnaire study of 3,069 women National Health and Nutrition Examination Study in the US.[59]

On the other hand, obesity is a risk factor for chronic migraine[60] and dietary-induced obesity may increase migraine by altering release of calcitonin gene-related peptide and increasing trigeminal sensitisation.[61] Obese women with migraine spent less time in physical activities than non-migraine sufferers, although the lower physical activities were not related to migraine characteristics.[62]

Menstrual Changes

Menses is perhaps the most common migraine trigger in women. It has been shown by previous studies that (1) menstruation was found to be the most significant hazard for migraine with an increase of migraine prevalence and persistence up to 96%;[63] (2) over half of women with migraine reported an increased rate of migraine related to menses;[64] (3) menstruation can trigger migraine, perhaps more so in those with aura;[65] and (4) migraine attacks during menses may be more severe, with reduced response to acute medication such as triptans.[66]

Estrogen withdrawal prior to menses is likely the cause of menstrual migraine and explains why migraine onset often commences prior to menstruation onset or on the first day.[67] For a significant minority of women, menstrual-related migraine may be more likely to occur towards the end of their cycle suggesting a relationship to blood loss or anemia.[68]

Weather

Multiple studies have considered the relationship between migraine or headache and environmental factors such as weather.

First of all, high altitude has been proven to be a trigger of headaches, especially during rapid ascents.[69] Several clinical studies have attempted to find correlations between migraine attacks and weather, focusing on variables such as barometric changes, lightning, temperature and precipitation. For example, Prince *et al.* (2004) reviewed 77 subjects with migraine and found 39/77 (50.6%) were sensitive to at least one weather factor;[70] Hoffman *et al.* (2011) reviewed the 12-month calendar data and found that six out of 20 subjects with migraine were significantly sensitive to weather changes, with lower temperature and higher humidity being associated with increased headache intensity.[71] A one-year calendar study in Japan found 18 of 28 patients had migraines related to weather changes, most commonly related to low barometric pressure.[72] For the migraine patients living at extreme latitudes such as the Arctic Circle, seasons and sunlight may trigger migraine.[73,74] In addition, a large-scale hierarchical clusters design study concluded that emergency department visits for headache are correlated to weather conditions as well as ambient air pollution.[75]

Sensory Stimuli

Visual, noise, olfactory and other sensory stimuli exacerbate migraine intensity and may cause migraine in vulnerable individuals. The thresholds of discomfort to stimuli of migraine patients are lower than non-migraineurs. This could be explained by a lack of habituation[76] and alteration in the processing of sensory stimuli.[77] However, it is difficult to sort out if sensory stimuli are triggers or if patients with migraine simply become more sensitive to stimuli in the premonitory phase prior to an attack.[78]

Stress and Sleep

Stress is perhaps the most common self-reported trigger of migraine, and many studies have been able to demonstrate a link between chronic stress, pain, migraine and catastrophic thinking.[79,80] Lipton *et al.* (2014) found that migraine is more likely to occur immediately after periods of reduced stress, suggesting that 'let-down' headache is probably more common than acute stress-related migraine.[81]

Poor sleep quality is commonly cited as a trigger for migraine, and in many patients with migraine, sleep helps treat an attack.[82] While sleep disturbances are a commonly reported trigger, diary studies do not consistently demonstrate it as a risk factor for migraine. Peris *et al.* (2017) found that restless sleep was a risk factor for migraine in only 25.2% of individuals.[56] Seidel *et al.* (2009) found that while sleep quality is reduced in migraine, rates of fatigue and daytime sleepiness are similar to controls, suggesting poor sleep is caused by migraine, not the other way around.[83]

Pathological Processes of Migraine

The pathological process of migraine is presented in two categories: aura and headaches.

Migraine Aura

Aura was explained by Lashley in the 1940s as the clinical manifestation of a spreading abnormality, which migrated over the visual cortex at a rate of three to five millimetres (mm) per minute.[84] Shortly thereafter, Leao (1944) described an electrophysiological event in experimental animal models that he called cortical spreading depression (CSD), in which mechanical or chemical stimulation of the cortical surface produced hyperexcitation followed by suppression that migrated over the cortical surface at a slow rate of three to four mm per minute.[85–87] In the 1950s, Milner proposed that CSD was the pathophysiological basis of migraine aura, based on a similar propagation rate and the migration of aura symptoms across neurovascular boundaries.[88]

Since the 1980s, researchers have been investing the physiological mechanisms of migraine aura through intra-arterial blood flow studies. It was shown that the regional cerebral blood flow (rCBF) decreases 17–35% in patients with migraine and typical aura.[89,90]

Such changes in rCBF were termed 'oligemia' because their magnitude was not great enough to be considered ischaemia and because the changes spread anteriorly across neurovascular boundaries.[89,90] The changes in rCBF typically normalised after an hour but could remain focally decreased and were not present in patients that had migraine without aura.[91,92]

The findings of cortical oligemia without ischaemia contralateral to the affected visual hemifield during visual aura were confirmed with other imaging modalities including positron emission tomography (15O-labelled water), functional magnetic resonance imaging (fMRI), and perfusion weighted imaging (PWI) in both spontaneous and provoked migraine attacks.[93,94] On the other hand, when migraine with aura patients did not have an aura or in patients with migraine without aura, perfusion deficits were not observed.[95]

In a blood oxygenation level-dependent (BOLD) fMRI study, it was reported that during exercise-induced visual auras there was a loss of cortical activation in the occipital lobe contralateral to the visual field in which the scotoma occurred that resolved after resolution of clinical symptoms.[96] These changes in BOLD activation expanded into the neighbouring cortex at a rate of 3.5 mm per minute and were consistent with BOLD fMRI findings observed in animal models of CSD.[96,97] Also, in the patients who experienced migraine attacks (both with and without aura) triggered by visual stimuli, both headache and visual symptoms were preceded by suppression of initial activation with slow propagation into the contiguous occipital cortex and accompanied by increased occipital cortex oxygenation.[98]

Migraine Headache

The absence of cortical 'oligemia' or cortical changes on functional imaging in migraine without aura resulted in a search for alternative theories to explain the origin of the headache phase of migraine. Activation of the trigeminocervical complex is the most likely explanation for the nociceptive component of migraine.[99–101] The ophthalmic branch of the trigeminal nerve innervates the dural and cranial vascular structures in the anterior and middle fossa, whereas the posterior fossa is innervated by the upper cervical roots.[101] Stimulation of these structures results in pain and increased neuronal activity in the respective locations.[101] The meningeal nerves also send branches and innervate both the pial surface and calvarial bones (through infiltration of the calvarial sutures).[102] There is convergence of input from the trigeminal and cervical afferents at the trigeminocervical complex (TCC).[101] Stimulation of the TCC can lead to activation of the trigeminovascular system with release of nociceptive and vasoactive peptides.[99–101]

The dilation of blood vessels observed during migraine headache does not appear to be extensive enough to cause pain.[99] Although a point of ongoing controversy, due to the fact that the blockade of some of the neuropeptides released during neurogenic plasma extravasation has not been effective in clinical trials of migraine,[101] the throbbing nature of pain in migraine headache is generally held to be related to peripheral sensitisation that occurs in the context of activation of the TCC.[99] The dilation of cerebral blood vessels during migraine headache is likely an epiphenomenon due to activation of the trigeminal-autonomic reflex and the literature does not support early vascular theories of the pathogenesis of migraine headache.[101] The development of migraine headache is likely related to the activation of nociceptive receptors on intracranial dural and vascular structures (at least partly due to the release of neuropeptides such as calcitonin gene-related peptide [CGRP]), activation of the thalamico-cortical networks and inhibition of descending cortical pain controlling pathways.[99,101]

Diagnosis of Migraine

The diagnostic criteria of migraine are detailed in the latest version of the International Classification of Headache Disorders introduced by the Headache Classification Committee of the International Headache Society.[1]

Migraine without Aura

Migraine without aura presents as a recurrent headache disorder manifesting in attacks lasting four to 72 hours. Typical characteristics of the headache are unilateral location, pulsating quality, moderate or severe intensity, aggravation by routine physical activity, and association with nausea and/or photophobia and phonophobia.[1]

The diagnostic criteria of migraine without aura are:

A. At least five attacks fulfilling criteria B–D;
B. Headache attacks lasting four to 72 hours (untreated or unsuccessfully treated);
C. Headache has at least two of the following four characteristics:

1. Unilateral location;
2. Pulsating quality;
3. Moderate or severe pain intensity;
4. Aggravation by, or causing avoidance of, routine physical activity (e.g. walking or climbing stairs).

D. During headache at least one of the following:

1. Nausea and/or vomiting;
2. Photophobia and phonophobia;

E. Not better accounted for by another ICHD-3 diagnosis.

It should be noted that, one or a few migraine attacks may be difficult to distinguish from symptomatic migraine-like attacks. Furthermore, the nature of a single or a few attacks may be difficult to understand. Therefore, at least five attacks are required.

Migraine with Aura

Migraine with aura presents headaches of recurrent attacks, lasting minutes, of unilateral fully reversible visual, sensory, or other central nervous system symptoms that usually develop gradually and are usually followed by headache and associated migraine symptoms.

The diagnostic criteria of migraine with aura are:

A. At least two attacks fulfilling criteria B and C;
B. One or more of the following fully reversible aura symptoms:

1. Visual;
2. Sensory;
3. Speech and/or language;
4. Motor;
5. Brainstem;
6. Retinal.

C. At least two of the following four characteristics:

1. At least one aura symptom spreads gradually over greater than five minutes, and/or two or more symptoms occur in succession;
2. Each individual aura symptom lasts five to 60 minutes;
3. At least one aura symptom is unilateral;
4. The aura is accompanied, or followed within 60 minutes, by headache.

D. Not better accounted for by another ICHD-3 diagnosis and transient ischaemic attack has been excluded.

The aura is the complex of neurological symptoms that occurs usually before the headache of migraine with aura, but it may begin after the pain phase has commenced or continue into the headache phase.[1]

Aura symptoms of these different types usually follow one another in succession, beginning with visual, then sensory, then aphasic symptoms, but the reverse and other orders have been noted. The accepted duration for most aura symptoms is one hour, but motor symptoms are often longer lasting. Patients often find it hard to describe their aura symptoms, in which case they should be instructed to time and record them prospectively. The clinical picture then becomes clearer. Common mistakes are incorrect reports of lateralisation, of sudden rather than gradual onset and of monocular rather than homonymous visual disturbances, as well as of duration of aura and mistaking sensory loss for weakness. After an initial consultation, use of an aura diary may clarify the diagnosis. In addition, some premonitory symptoms may begin hours, or a day or two, before the other symptoms of a migraine attack (with or without aura). They include various combinations of fatigue, difficulty in concentrating, neck stiffness, sensitivity to light and/or sound, nausea, blurred vision, yawning and pallor. These symptoms should not be classified as aura of migraine. Also, it is suggested to avoid using the terms 'prodrome' and 'warning symptoms' to describe these symptoms because they are often mistakenly used to include aura.[1]

Management of Migraine

Migraine is often underdiagnosed, misdiagnosed and undertreated in both primary and secondary care.[33] In recent years there have been advances in the diagnosis and treatment of migraine. There are new therapies for both acute and preventative treatment of patients with migraine.

Patient Perspective

Patients may have different perspectives on health care processes and outcomes from those of health care professionals. The involvement of patients in guideline development is therefore important to ensure that guidelines reflect their needs and concerns, and address issues that matter to them.[103]

Common concerns raised by patient groups and through research include the following:

- Quality-of-life issues around coping with pain, sleep disturbance and restriction on daily activities, education, working and social life, and the impact it has on the family;

- Concerns around side effects of pharmacological therapies, medication overuse and feeling dependent on prophylactic therapies;
- The need for clear information on the use of preventer medication.

Pharmacologic Treatments

The pharmacologic treatments presented in this section are based on the recommendations of pharmacological management of migraine guidelines developed by the Scottish Intercollegiate Guidelines Network (SIGN).[103]

Treatment for Patients with Acute Migraine

Acute treatment is used either to abort an attack of migraine or to significantly reduce the severity of the headache and other symptoms. Acute treatment should be taken as soon as the patient knows they are developing a migraine headache.[103] In patients who have aura, it is recommended that triptans are taken at the start of the headache and not at the start of the aura (unless the aura and headache start at the same time).[103] It is given once, with the option of repeating after two hours (with the same or different treatment) if there is an inadequate response.

Non-steroidal Anti-inflammatory Drugs

Aspirin (900 mg) is recommended as first-line treatment for patients with acute migraine. Aspirin, in doses for migraine, is not an analgesic of choice during pregnancy and should not be used in the third trimester of pregnancy.[104,105] Ibuprofen (400 mg) is also recommended as first-line treatment for patients with acute migraine. If ineffective, the dose should be increased to 600 mg.

Paracetamol

Paracetamol (1,000 mg) can be considered for treatment of patients with acute migraine who are unable to take other acute therapies. Due to its safety profile, paracetamol is the first choice for the short-term relief of mild to moderate headache during any trimester of pregnancy.[106,107]

Antiemetics

Metoclopramide (10 mg) or prochlorperazine (10 mg) can be considered in the treatment of headache in patients with acute migraine when they presenting with migraine-associated symptoms of nausea or vomiting. They can be used either as an oral form or parenteral form depending on presentation and setting. Metoclopramide is associated with the risk of extrapyramidal side effects; therefore it sholud be used with caution.

Triptans

Triptans are recommended as the first-line treatment for patients with acute migraine. The first choice is sumatriptan (50–100 mg); others can be used when sumatriptan fails. Nasal zolmitriptan or subcutaneous sumatriptan should be considered for patients who present severe acute migraine or early vomiting. Triptans are recommended for the treatment of patients with acute migraine associated with menstruation. Sumatriptan can be considered for treatment of acute migraine in pregnant women in all stages of pregnancy. The risks associated with use should be discussed before commencing treatment.

Combined Therapies

Combination therapy using sumatriptan (50–85 mg) and naproxen (500 mg) should be considered for the treatment of patients with acute migraine.

Pharmacological Prevention of Episodic Migraine

Migraine causes considerable impact on quality of life and daily function. Modest improvements in the frequency or severity of migraine headaches may benefit the patients significantly. Therefore, a reduction in migraine headache severity and/or frequency of

30–50% is regarded as successful treatment effects in clinical studies. The decision about when to start migraine prophylaxis should be guided by establishing the impact of migraine on each patient, rather than just focusing on the absolute number of headaches or migraines per month. For example, a few severe incapacitating migraines per month may warrant prophylactic treatment, whereas more frequent but milder migraines that have little impact on daily function may not require treatment. It should be noted that, overusing acute medication can limit the effectiveness of preventative medication and medication overuse should also be assessed and addressed.[108]

Prophylactic treatment should be used for at least three months at the maximum tolerated dose before determining whether it is effective or not. In many patients, prophylactic medication can be successfully phased out and the need for ongoing prophylaxis should be considered after six to 12 months.[109] Choosing which medication to use first is dependent on evidence of effectiveness, patient comorbidities, other risk factors, drug interactions and patient preference. It is important to ensure adequate contraception whilst on preventative therapies as some have risks of teratogenicity and others may impact on unborn babies.

Given that migraine without aura often improves during pregnancy, women should aim to stop migraine prophylactic treatments before pregnancy.[37] Migraine with aura often continues unchanged.[37] Before commencing treatment, potential harmful effects of therapies need to be discussed with women who are, or may become, pregnant. No evidence was identified on which to base recommendations on preventative treatments for women during pregnancy.

Below listed are the common prophylactic treatment medication for episodic migraine.[103]

Beta Blockers

Propranolol (80–160 mg daily) is recommended as a first-line prophylactic treatment for patients with episodic or chronic migraine.

Topiramate

Topiramate (50–100 mg daily) is recommended as a prophylactic treatment for patients with episodic or chronic migraine. Before commencing treatment, women who may become pregnant should be advised of the associated risks of topiramate during pregnancy, the need to use effective contraception, and the need to seek further advice on migraine prophylaxis if pregnant or planning a pregnancy.

Tricyclic Antidepressants

Amitriptyline (25–150 mg at night) should be considered as a prophylactic treatment for patients with episodic or chronic migraine. In patients who cannot tolerate amitriptyline, a less sedating tricyclic antidepressant should be considered.

Candesartan

Candesartan (16 mg daily) can be considered as a prophylactic treatment for patients with episodic or chronic migraine.

Sodium Valproate

Sodium valproate (400–1,500 mg daily) can be considered as a prophylactic treatment for patients with episodic or chronic migraine.

Prescribers should be aware that sodium valproate is associated with an increased risk of foetal malformations and poorer cognitive outcomes in children exposed to valproate *in utero*. For women who may become pregnant, sodium valproate should only be considered as a prophylactic treatment when:

- Other treatment options have been exhausted;
- Patients are using adequate contraception.

Before commencing treatment, women should be informed of:

- The risks associated with taking sodium valproate during pregnancy;
- The risk that potentially harmful exposure to sodium valproate may occur before a woman is aware she is pregnant;

- The need to use effective contraception;
- The need to seek further advice on migraine prophylaxis if pregnant or planning a pregnancy.

Calcium Channel Blockers

Flunarizine (10 mg daily) should be considered as a prophylactic treatment for patients with episodic or chronic migraine.

Pizotifen

There is insufficient evidence to support a recommendation, but pizotifen is a well-established therapy which is widely used.[103]

Triptans

Frovatriptan (2.5 mg twice daily) should be considered as a prophylactic treatment in women with perimenstrual migraine from two days before, until three days after, bleeding starts. Zolmitriptan (2.5 mg three times daily) or naratriptan (2.5 mg twice daily) can be considered as alternatives to frovatriptan as prophylactic treatment in women with perimenstrual migraine from two days before, until three days after, bleeding starts.

Women with menstrual-related migraine, who are using triptans at other times of the month, should be advised that additional perimenstrual prophylaxis increases the risk of developing medication overuse headache.

Non-pharmacological Devices for Migraine Therapies

Devices may offer an alternative, or an addition, to pharmacological therapies but few trials have been conducted on their efficacy and safety.[110,111] These are:

- Vagus nerve stimulation;
- Transcutaneous supraorbital nerve stimulation;
- Transcranial magnetic stimulation.

Other Management for Migraine

Lifestyle factors may trigger, or influence, the presence of individual migraine attacks, so non-pharmaceutical approaches become a key component to effective migraine prevention and management.

Avoiding Lifestyle Triggers

Unhealthy and irregular lifestyle factors may lower the headache threshold, or even trigger individual migraine attacks. Targeting and treating lifestyle factors seem quite simple, but when done effectively can have profound positive effects on migraine frequency.[112] Consistent meals/hydration and appropriate sleep hygiene can provide the stability needed to decrease the likelihood of migraines. Lifestyle factors important in migraine prevention include:

- Regularly scheduled meals — avoid missing or delaying meal times;
- Routine hydration with non-caffeinated beverages throughout the day;
- Consistent sleep schedule every night of the week, including weekends.

Focusing on lifestyle triggers as the prevention for migraine appeals to patients and clinicians wanting to promote wellness and reduce medication use. Successful treatment of migraine, like many other chronic illnesses, necessitates involving patients in their care, encouraging proactive behaviours and using a 'patient-centred care' approach.[113]

However, focusing extensively on migraine triggers may have negative consequences: (1) patients may feel 'blamed' or stigmatised for having a migraine; (2) migraine triggers may be impossible to figure out, especially in those with very frequent or infrequent attacks; (3) the triggers may not be avoidable; (4) focusing on triggers can increase anxiety or lead to anticipation of attacks; and (5) it does not address the underlying cause of the disorder. An excessive focus on avoiding triggers may in fact be harmful. Avoiding stress in chronic pain is less effective than coping or adaptive strategies and may lead to anxiety, reduced physical activity, increased disability and catastrophic thinking.[114,115] A recent study by Martin *et al.* (2014) found the standard advice to avoid triggers was not effective in reducing migraine, compared to a waitlist control group, and less effective than cognitive therapy or a 'learning to cope with triggers' approach.[116]

With this in mind, here are a few strategies to utilise when advising patients with migraine on triggers[51]:

1. Keep a headache journal or calendar;
2. Focus on healthy lifestyle choices rather than trigger avoidance;
3. Recognise 'cephalgiaphobia' and treat it aggressively;
4. For frequent attacks, recommend prevention.

Mind/Body Practices

Stress is the number one reported trigger for migraines. Treatments that target stress may be particularly beneficial in decreasing migraine frequency and in building additional coping behaviours[112]:

- Cognitive behavioural therapy, including stress management and coping skills;
- Biofeedback (electromyographic and thermal with relaxation);
- Relaxation training.

Complementary and Alternative Medicine Therapies

Pharmaceutical options have many limitations, such as side effects and limited efficacy, and may not be suitable for pregnant and breast-feeding women. These limitations may explain why up to 82% of patients seek complementary and alternative medicines to manage their migraine.[112,117]

Acupuncture has been extensively researched as the management for migraine prevention. There is growing evidence that acupuncture is just as effective and has fewer side effects than many of the standard pharmaceutical agents that are currently used.[118]

A recently published overview of systematic reviews concluded that acupuncture on treating migraine has the advantage for pain improvement and safety, but the quality of systematic review or meta-analysis of acupuncture for migraine remains to be improved.[119] Previously published systematic reviews showed that oral Chinese herbal medicine was more effective than placebo or conventional pharmacotherapies for migraine prophylactic treatment; however, the results remain uncertain due to their limitations of included studies.[120–123] Massage is not a treatment typically recommended for use in migraine; for those patients who can afford it and find symptomatic relief, it may be helpful.[112] Other herbs, vitamins and minerals may help prevent headaches. Although considered 'natural', side effects can occur.[112]

Prognosis of Migraine

Most patients with episodic migraine do well with treatment. However, 2.5% of people with episodic migraine each year develop chronic migraine.[124] In population-based surveys the frequency of migraine headaches decreases with age.[125] The prognosis is guarded for patients who have developed complications of migraine, or who have comorbidities or a longstanding history of medication overuse. In these cases, expectations for improvement should be modest, and the goals of treatment should shift from elimination of pain to improvement in function.[126] A summary of this chapter can be seen in Table 1.1.

Table 1.1. Chapter Summary

Definition	• Primary headache disorder with recurrent episodes of headache manifesting in attacks lasting from four to 72 hours.
Main characteristics	• Typical characteristics of the headache are unilateral location, pulsating quality, moderate or severe intensity, aggravated by routine physical activity and association with nausea, photophobia or phonophobia, or any combination of all these three.

(Continued)

Table 1.1.   (*Continued*)

Diagnosis	• Clinical features and associated symptoms; • Physical examination; • Lab examination, EEG, TCD, brain CT/MRI scans to exclude secondary headache disorders.
Management	• Patient's education: A proper goal, healthy lifestyle, headache diary; • Non-pharmacologic treatment; • Pharmacologic treatments.
Pharmacological management	• Acute management: NSAIDs, paracetamol, triptans, antiemetics, combined therapies; • Prevention treatment: beta blockers, topiramate, tricyclic antidepressants, candesartan, sodium valproate, calcium channel blockers, pizotifen, botulinum toxin A.

Abbreviations: CT, computerised tomography; EEG, electroencephalography; MRI, magnetic resonance imaging; NSAIDs, non-steroidal anti-inflammatory drugs; TCD, transcranial Doppler.

References

1. Headache Classification Committee of the International Headache Society (IHS). (2018) The International Classification of Headache Disorders, 3rd ed. *Cephalalgia* **38(1):** 1–211.
2. Lipton RB, Silberstein SD. (2015) Episodic and chronic migraine headache: Breaking down barriers to optimal treatment and prevention. *Headache* **55(Suppl 2):** 103–122; quiz 123–126.
3. Manzoni GC, Farina S, Lanfranchi M, Solari A. (1985) Classic migraine: Clinical findings in 164 patients. *Eur Neurol* **24(3):** 163–169.
4. Eriksen MK, Thomsen LL, Andersen I, *et al.* (2004) Clinical characteristics of 362 patients with familial migraine with aura. *Cephalalgia* **24(7):** 564–575.
5. Bana DS, Graham JR. (1986) Observations on prodromes of classic migraine in a headache clinic population. *Headache* **26(5):** 216–219.
6. Russell MB, Olesen J. (1996) A nosographic analysis of the migraine aura in a general population. *Brain* **119(2):** 355–361.
7. Cutrer FM, Huerter K. (2007) Migraine aura. *Neurologist* **13(3):** 118–125.

8. Bradshaw P, Parsons M. (1965) Hemiplegic migraine, a clinical study. *Q J Med* **34**: 65–85.
9. Lykke Thomsen L, Kirchmann Eriksen M, Faerch Romer S, *et al.* (2002) An epidemiological survey of hemiplegic migraine. *Cephalalgia* **22(5)**: 361–375.
10. Kirchmann M, Thomsen LL, Olesen J. (2006) Basilar-type migraine: Clinical, epidemiologic and genetic features. *Neurology* **66(6)**: 880–886.
11. Kirchmann M. (2006) Migraine with aura: New understanding from clinical epidemiologic studies. *Curr Opin Neurol* **19(3)**: 286–293.
12. Kaniecki RG. (2009) Basilar-type migraine. *Curr Pain Headache Rep* **13(3)**: 217–220.
13. Ziegler DK, Hassanein RS. (1990) Specific headache phenomena: Their frequency and coincidence. *Headache* **30(3)**: 152–156.
14. Queiroz LP, Rapoport AM, Weeks RE, *et al.* (1997) Characteristics of migraine visual aura. *Headache* **37(3)**: 137–141.
15. Queiroz LP, Friedman DI, Rapoport AM, Purdy RA. (2011) Characteristics of migraine visual aura in Southern Brazil and Northern USA. *Cephalalgia* **31(16)**: 1652–1658.
16. Russell MB, Iversen HK, Olesen J. (1994) Improved description of the migraine aura by a diagnostic aura diary. *Cephalalgia* **14(2)**: 107–117.
17. Hupp SL, Kline LB, Corbett JJ. (1989) Visual disturbances of migraine. *Surv Ophthalmol* **33(4)**: 221–236.
18. Russo A, Marcelli V, Esposito F, *et al.* (2014) Abnormal thalamic function in patients with vestibular migraine. *Neurology* **82(23)**: 2120–2126.
19. Espinosa-Sanchez JM, Lopez-Escamez JA. (2015) New insights into pathophysiology of vestibular migraine. *Front Neurol* **6**: 12.
20. Teggi R, Colombo B, Rocca MA, *et al.* (2016) A review of recent literature on functional MRI and personal experience in two cases of definite vestibular migraine. *Neurol Sci* **37(9)**: 1399–1402.
21. Morrison DP. (1990) Abnormal perceptual experiences in migraine. *Cephalalgia* **10(6)**: 273–277.
22. Coleman ER, Grosberg BM, Robbins MS. (2011) Olfactory hallucinations in primary headache disorders: Case series and literature review. *Cephalalgia* **31(14)**: 1477–1489.
23. Miller EE, Grosberg BM, Crystal SC, Robbins MS. (2015) Auditory hallucinations associated with migraine: Case series and literature review. *Cephalalgia* **35(10)**: 923–930.

24. Mainardi F, Rapoport A, Zanchin G, Maggioni F. (2016) Scent of aura? Clinical features of olfactory hallucinations during a migraine attack (OHM). *Cephalalgia* **37(2):** 154–160.

25. Agostoni E, Aliprandi A. (2006) The complications of migraine with aura. *Neurol Sci* **27(Suppl 2):** S91–S95.

26. Lauritzen M, Strong AJ. (2017) 'Spreading depression of Leao' and its emerging relevance to acute brain injury in humans. *J Cereb Blood Flow Metab* **37(5):** 1553–1570.

27. Nye BL, Thadani VM. (2015) Migraine and epilepsy: Review of the literature. *Headache* **55(3):** 359–380.

28. Wei Y, Ullah G, Schiff SJ. (2014) Unification of neuronal spikes, seizures, and spreading depression. *J Neurosci* **34(35):** 11733–11743.

29. Dreier JP, Major S, Pannek HW, *et al.* (2012) Spreading convulsions, spreading depolarization and epileptogenesis in human cerebral cortex. *Brain* **135(Pt 1):** 259–275.

30. Steiner TJ, Stovner LJ, Birbeck GL. (2013) Migraine: The seventh disabler. *J Headache Pain* **14(1):** 1.

31. GBD 2017 Disease and Injury Incidence and Prevalence Collaborators. (2018) Global, regional, and national incidence, prevalence, and years lived with disability for 354 diseases and injuries for 195 countries and territories, 1990–2017: A systematic analysis for the Global Burden of Disease Study 2017. *Lancet* **392(10159):** 1789–1858.

32. Schreiber CP, Hutchinson S, Webster CJ, *et al.* (2004) Prevalence of migraine in patients with a history of selfreported or physician-diagnosed 'sinus' headache. *Arch Intern Med* **164(16):** 1769–1772.

33. Tepper SJ, Dahlof CG, Dowson A, *et al.* (2004) Prevalence and diagnosis of migraine in patients consulting their physician with a complaint of headache: Data from the Landmark Study. *Headache* **44(9):** 856–864.

34. Buse DC, Loder EW, Gorman JA, *et al.* (2013) Sex differences in the prevalence, symptoms and associated features of migraine, probable migraine and other severe headache: Results of the American migraine prevalence and prevention (AMPP) study. *Headache* **53(8):** 1278–1299.

35. Vetvik KG, MacGregor EA. (2017) Sex differences in the epidemiology, clinical features and pathophysiology of migraine. *Lancet Neurol* **16(1):** 76–87.

36. MacGregor EA. (2007) Migraine, the menopause and hormone replacement therapy: A clinical review. *J Fam Plann Reprod Health Care* **33(4):** 245–249.

37. Stewart WF, Roy J, Lipton RB. (2013) Migraine prevalence, socioeconomic status, and social causation. *Neurology* **81(11):** 948–955.

38. Manzoni GC, Stovner LJ. (2010) Epidemiology of headache. *Handb Clin Neurol* **97:** 3–22.

39. Russell MB, Rasmussen BK, Thorvaldsen P, Olesen J. (1995) Prevalence and sex-ratio of the subtypes of migraine. *Int J Epidemiol* **24(3):** 612–618.

40. Stewart WF, Linet MS, Celentano DD, *et al.* (1991) Age- and sex-specific incidence rates of migraine with and without visual aura. *Am J Epidemiol* **134(10):** 1111–1120.

41. Lipton RB, Bigal ME, Diamond M, *et al.* (2007) Migraine prevalence, disease burden, and the need for preventive therapy. *Neurology* **68(5):** 343–349.

42. Vos T, Flaxman AD, Naghavi M, *et al.* (2012) Years lived with disability (YLD) for 1160 sequelae of 289 diseases and injuries 1990–2010: A systematic analysis for the Global Burden of Disease Study 2010. *Lancet* **380(9859):** 2163–2196.

43. Steiner TJ, Stovner LJ, Vos T. (2016) GBD 2015: Migraine is the third cause of disability in under 50s. *J Headache Pain* **17(1):** 104.

44. Hu XH, Markson LE, Lipton RB, *et al.* (1999) Burden of migraine in the United States: Disability and economic costs. *Arch Intern Med* **159(8):** 813–818.

45. Edmeads J, Mackell JA. (2002) The economic impact of migraine: An analysis of direct and indirect costs. *Headache* **42(6):** 501–509.

46. Lambert J, Carides GW, Meloche JP, *et al.* (2002) Impact of migraine symptoms on health care use and work loss in Canada in patients randomly assigned in a phase III clinical trial. *Can J Clin Pharmacol* **9(3):** 158–164.

47. Stokes M, Becker WJ, Lipton RB, *et al.* (2011) Cost of health care among patients with chronic and episodic migraine in Canada and the USA: Results from the International Burden of Migraine Study (IBMS). *Headache* **51(7):** 1058–1077.

48. All-Party Parliamentary Group on Primary Headache Disorders (APPGPHD). (2010) Headache disorders: Not respected, not resourced: A report of the all-party parliamentary group on primary headache disorders (APPGPHD). Available from: https://www.migrainetrust.org/wp-content/uploads/2015/12/2010Mar-APPGPHD_REPORT_Headache_Disorders-NotRespNotReso.pdf.

49. Deloitte Access Economics Report. (2018) Migraine in Australia Whitepaper. Prepared for Novartis Australia. Available from: https://www2.deloitte.com/au/en/pages/economics/articles/migraine-australia-whitepaper.html.

50. 中华医学会疼痛学分会头面痛学组. (2016) 中国偏头痛防治指南. 中国疼痛医学杂志. **22(10)**.

51. Marmura MJ. (2018) Triggers, protectors, and predictors in episodic migraine. *Curr Pain Headache Rep* **22(12):** 81.

52. Becker WJ. (2013) The premonitory phase of migraine and migraine management. *Cephalalgia* **33(13):** 1117–1121.

53. Schoonman GG, Evers DJ, Terwindt GM, *et al.* (2006) The prevalence of premonitory symptoms in migraine: A questionnaire study in 461 patients. *Cephalalgia* **26(10):** 1209–1213.

54. Maniyar FH, Sprenger T, Schankin C, Goadsby PJ. (2014) Photic hypersensitivity in the premonitory phase of migraine: A positron emission tomography study. *Eur J Neurol* **21(9):** 1178–1183.

55. Holm JE, Bury L, Suda KT. (1996) The relationship between stress, headache, and the menstrual cycle in young female migraineurs. *Headache* **36(9):** 531–537.

56. Peris F, Donoghue S, Torres F, *et al.* (2017) Towards improved migraine management: Determining potential trigger factors in individual patients. *Cephalalgia* **37(5):** 452–463.

57. Monro J, Brostoff J, Carini C, Zilkha K. (1980) Food allergy in migraine: Study of dietary exclusion and RAST. *Lancet* **2(8184):** 1–4.

58. Sensenig J, Johnson M, Staverosky T. (2001) Treatment of migraine with targeted nutrition focused on improved assimilation and elimination. *Altern Med Rev* **6(5):** 488–494.

59. Evans EW, Lipton RB, Peterlin BL, *et al.* (2015) Dietary intake patterns and diet quality in a nationally representative sample of women with and without severe headache or migraine. *Headache* **55(4):** 550–561.

60. Bigal ME, Lipton RB. (2006) Obesity is a risk factor for transformed migraine but not chronic tension-type headache. *Neurology* **67(2):** 252–257.

61. Marics B, Peitl B, Varga A, *et al.* (2017) Diet-induced obesity alters dural CGRP release and potentiates TRPA1-mediated trigeminovascular responses. *Cephalalgia.* **37(6):** 581–591.

62. Bond DS, Thomas JG, O'Leary KC, *et al.* (2015) Objectively measured physical activity in obese women with and without migraine. *Cephalalgia* **35(10):** 886–893.

63. Wober C, Brannath W, Schmidt K, *et al.* (2007) Prospective analysis of factors related to migraine attacks: The PAMINA study. *Cephalalgia* **27(4):** 304–314.

64. Karli N, Baykan B, Ertas M, *et al.* (2012) Impact of sex hormonal changes on tension-type headache and migraine: A cross-sectional population-based survey in 2,600 women. *J Headache Pain* **13(7):** 557–565.

65. Salhofer-Polanyi S, Frantal S, Brannath W, *et al.* (2012) Prospective analysis of factors related to migraine aura: The PAMINA study. *Headache* **52(8):** 1236–1245.

66. Bhambri R, Martin VT, Abdulsattar Y, *et al.* (2014) Comparing the efficacy of eletriptan for migraine in women during menstrual and non-menstrual time periods: A pooled analysis of randomized controlled trials. *Headache* **54(2):** 343–354.

67. Loder EW. (2006) Menstrual migraine: Pathophysiology, diagnosis and impact. *Headache* **46(Suppl 2):** S55–S60.

68. Calhoun AH, Gill N. (2017) Presenting a new, non-hormonally mediated cyclic headache in women: End-menstrual migraine. *Headache* **57(1):** 17–20.

69. Marmura MJ, Hernandez PB. (2015) High-altitude headache. *Curr Pain Headache Rep* **19(5):** 483.

70. Prince PB, Rapoport AM, Sheftell FD, *et al.* (2004) The effect of weather on headache. *Headache* **44(6):** 596–602.

71. Hoffmann J, Lo H, Neeb L, *et al.* (2011) Weather sensitivity in migraineurs. *J Neurol* **258(4):** 596–602.

72. Kimoto K, Aiba S, Takashima R, *et al.* (2011) Influence of barometric pressure in patients with migraine headache. *Intern Med* **50(18):** 1923–1928.

73. Ivar BS, Hindberg K, Bashari H, *et al.* (2011) Sun-induced migraine attacks in an Arctic population. *Cephalalgia* **31(9):** 992–998.

74. Salvesen R, Bekkelund SI. (2000) Migraine, as compared to other headaches, is worse during midnight-sun summer than during polar night. A questionnaire study in an Arctic population. *Headache* **40(10):** 824–829.

75. Szyszkowicz M. (2008) Migraine, as compared to other headaches, is worse during midnight-sun summer than during polar night. A questionnaire study in an Arctic population. *Headache.* **48(3):** 417–423.

76. Gierse-Plogmeier B, Colak-Ekici R, Wolowski A, *et al.* (2009) Differences in trigeminal and peripheral electrical pain perception in women with and without migraine. *J Headache Pain* **10(4):** 249–254.

77. Schwedt TJ, Chong CD, Chiang CC, *et al.* (2014) Enhanced pain-induced activity of pain-processing regions in a case-control study of episodic migraine. *Cephalalgia* **34(12):** 947–958.

78. Schulte LH, Jurgens TP, May A. (2015) Photo-, osmo- and phonophobia in the premonitory phase of migraine: Mistaking symptoms for triggers? *J Headache Pain* **16:** 14.

79. Meng ID, Cao L. (2007) From migraine to chronic daily headache: The biological basis of headache transformation. *Headache* **47(8):** 1251–1258.

80. Kunz M, Chatelle C, Lautenbacher S, Rainville P. (2008) The relation between catastrophizing and facial responsiveness to pain. *Pain* **140(1):** 127–134.

81. Lipton RB, Buse DC, Hall CB, *et al.* (2014) Reduction in perceived stress as a migraine trigger: Testing the 'let-down headache' hypothesis. *Neurology* **82(16):** 1395–1401.

82. Bigal ME, Hargreaves RJ. (2013) Why does sleep stop migraine? *Curr Pain Headache Rep* **17(10):** 369.

83. Seidel S, Hartl T, Weber M, *et al.* (2009) Quality of sleep, fatigue and daytime sleepiness in migraine: A controlled study. *Cephalalgia* **29(6):** 662–669.

84. Lashley KS. (1941) Patterns of cerebral integration indicated by the scotomas of migraine. *Arch Neurol Psychiatry* **46(2):** 259–264.

85. Leao AA. (1944) Spreading depression of activity in the cerebral cortex. *J Neurophysiol* **7:** 359–390.

86. Leao AA. (1947) Further observations on the spreading depression of activity in the cerebral cortex. *J Neurophysiol* **10:** 409–414.

87. Leao AA. (1951) The slow voltage variation of cortical spreading depression of activity. *Electroencephalogr Clin Neurophysiol* **3:** 315–321.

88. Milner PM. (1958) Note on a possible correspondence between the scotomas of migraine and spreading depression of Leao. *Electroencephalogr Clin Neurophysiol* **10:** 705.

89. Lauritzen M, Skyhoj Olsen T, Lassen NA, Paulson OB. (1983) Changes in regional cerebral blood flow during the course of classic migraine attacks. *Ann Neurol* **13(6):** 633–641.

90. Olesen J, Larsen B, Lauritzen M. (1981) Focal hyperemia followed by spreading oligemia and impaired activation of rCBF in classic migraine. *Ann Neurol.* **9(4):** 344–352.

91. Olesen J, Friberg L, Olsen TS, *et al.* (1990) Timing and topography of cerebral blood flow, aura, and headache during migraine attacks. *Ann Neurol.* **28(6):** 791–798.

92. Lauritzen M, Olesen J. (1984) Regional cerebral blood flow during migraine attacks by Xenon-133 inhalation and emission tomography. *Brain* **107:** 447–461.

93. Woods RP, Iacoboni M, Mazziotta JC. (1994) Brief report: Bilateral spreading cerebral hypoperfusion during spontaneous migraine headache. *N Engl J Med* **331(25):** 1689–1692.

94. Cutrer FM, Sorensen AG, Weisskoff RM, *et al.* (1998) Perfusion weighted imaging defects during spontaneous migrainous aura. *Ann Neurol* **43(1):** 25–31.

95. Sanchez del Rio M, Bakker D, Wu O, *et al.* (1999) Perfusion weighted imaging during migraine: Spontaneous visual aura and headache. *Cephalalgia* **19(8):** 701–707.

96. Hadjikhani N, Sanchez Del Rio M, Wu O, *et al.* (2001) Mechanisms of migraine aura revealed by functional MRI in human visual cortex. *Proc Natl Acad Sci U S A* **98(8):** 4687–4692.

97. James MF, Smith MI, Bockhorst KH, *et al.* (1999) Cortical spreading depression in the gyrencephalic feline brain studied by magnetic resonance imaging. *J Physiol* **519(Pt 2):** 415–425.

98. Cao Y, Welch KM, Aurora S, Vikingstad EM. (1999) Functional MRI-BOLD of visually triggered headache in patients with migraine. *Arch Neurol* **56(5):** 548–554.

99. Noseda R, Burstein R. (2013) Migraine pathophysiology: Anatomy of the trigeminovascular pathway and associated neurological symptoms, CSD, sensitization and modulation of pain. *Pain* **154(Suppl 1):** 1–21.

100. Buzzi MG, Moskowitz MA. (2005) The pathophysiology of migraine: Year 2005. *J Headache Pain* **6(3):** 105–111.

101. Goadsby PJ, Charbit AR, Andreou AP, *et al.* (2009) Neurobiology of migraine. *Neuroscience* **161(2):** 327–341.

102. Kosaras B, Jakubowski M, Kainz V, Burstein R. (2009) Sensory innervation of the calvarial bones of the mouse. *J Comp Neurol* **515(3):** 331–348.

103. Scottish Intercollegiate Guidelines Network (SIGN). (2018) Pharmacological management of migraine (SIGN publication no. 155). Available from: http://www.sign.ac.uk.

104. British Association for the Study of Headache (BASH). (2010) Guidelines for all healthcare professionals in the diagnosis and management of migraine, tension-type, cluster and medication-overuse headache. Available from: http://www.bash.org.uk/wp-content/uploads/2012/07/10102-BASH-Guidelines-update-2_v5-1-indd.pdf.

105. Joint Formulary Committee. Guidance on prescribing. In: British National Formulary (online) London: BMJ Group and Pharmaceutical Press. Available from: https://www.medicinescomplete.com/mc/bnf/current/PHP97234-guidance-on-prescribing.htm.

106. Briggs G, Freeman R, Towers C, Forinash A. (2017) *Drugs in Pregnancy and Lactation: A Reference Guide to Fetal and Neonatal Risk*, 11th ed. Lippincott Williams & Wilkins, PA.

107. Schaefer C, Peters PWJ, RK M. (2014) *Drugs during Pregnancy and Lactation*, 3rd ed. Academic Press, London.

108. Zeeberg P, Olesen J, Jensen R. (2006) Discontinuation of medication overuse in headache patients: Recovery of therapeutic responsiveness. *Cephalalgia* **26(10):** 1192–1198.

109. Diener HC, Agosti R, Allais G, *et al.* (2007) Cessation versus continuation of 6-month migraine preventive therapy with topiramate (PROMPT): A randomised, double-blind, placebo-controlled trial. *Lancet Neurol* **6(12):** 1054–1062.

110. National Institute for Health and Care Excellence (NICE). (2014) Transcranial magnetic stimulation for treating and preventing migraine (Interventional procedures guidance no. 477). Available from: https://www.nice.org.uk/guidance/ipg477.

111. National Institute for Health and Care Excellence (NICE). (2016) Transcutaneous stimulation of the cervical branch of the vagus nerve for cluster headache and migraine (Interventional procedures guidance no. 552). Available from: https://www.nice.org.uk/guidance/ipg552/resources/transcutaneous-stimulation-of-thecervical-branch-of-the-vagus-nerve-for-cluster-headache-andmigraine-1899871983899845.

112. Wells RE, Baute V, Wahbeh H. (2017) Complementary and Integrative Medicine for Neurologic Conditions. *Med Clin North Am* **101(5):** 881–893.

113. Barry MJ, Edgman-Levitan S. (2012) Shared decision making: Pinnacle of patient-centered care. *N Engl J Med* **366(9):** 780–781.

114. Ramirez-Maestre C, Esteve R, Lopez-Martinez A. (2014) Fear-avoidance, pain acceptance and adjustment to chronic pain: A cross-sectional study on a sample of 686 patients with chronic spinal pain. *Ann Behav Med* **48(3):** 402–410.

115. Volders S, Boddez Y, De Peuter S, *et al.* (2015) Avoidance behavior in chronic pain research: A cold case revisited. *Behav Res Ther* **64:** 31–37.

116. Martin PR, Reece J, Callan M, *et al.* (2014) Behavioral management of the triggers of recurrent headache: A randomized controlled trial. *Behav Res Ther* **61:** 1–11.

117. Adams J, Barbery G, Lui CW. (2013) Complementary and alternative medicine use for headache and migraine: A critical review of the literature. *Headache* **53(3):** 459–473.

118. Zhang N, Houle T, Hindiyeh N, Aurora SK. (2020) Systematic review: Acupuncture vs standard pharmacological therapy for migraine prevention. *Headache* **60(2):** 309–317.

119. Zhang XT, Li XY, Zhao C, *et al.* (2019) An overview of systematic reviews of randomized controlled trials on acupuncture treating migraine. *Pain Res Manag* **2019:** 5930627.

120. Xia W, Zhu M, Zhang Z, *et al.* (2013) Effect of *Tianshu* capsule in treatment of migraine: A meta-analysis of randomized control trials. *J Tradit Chin Med* **33(1):** 9–14.

121. Zhou L, Chen P, Liu L, *et al.* (2013) Systematic review and meta-analysis of traditional Chinese medicine in the treatment of migraines. *Am J Chin Med.* **41(5):** 1011–1025.

122. Xiao Y, Yuan L, Liu Y, *et al.* (2015) Traditional Chinese patent medicine for prophylactic treatment of migraine: A meta-analysis of randomized, double-blind, placebo-controlled trials. *Eur J Neurol* **22(2):** 361–368.

123. Shan CS, Xu QQ, Shi YH, *et al.* (2008) Chuanxiong formulae for migraine: A systematic review and meta-analysis of high-quality randomized controlled trials. *Front Pharmacol* **9:** 589.

124. Bigal ME, Serrano D, Buse D, *et al.* (2008) Acute migraine medications and evolution from epoisodic to chronic migraine: A longitudinal population-based study. *Headache* **48(8):** 1157–1168.

125. Lipton RB, Bigal ME. (2005) The epidemiology of migraine. *Am J Med* **118(Suppl 1):** 3S–10S.

126. Lipton RB, Silberstein SD, Saper JR, *et al.* (2003) Why headache treatment fails. *Neurology* **60(7):** 1064–1070.

2

Migraine in Chinese Medicine

OVERVIEW

Migraine has been recorded in classical Chinese medicine literature under disease names such as *tou feng* 头风, *shou feng* 首风, *nao feng* 脑风, *tou tong* 头痛 and *pian tou feng* 偏头风. The symptoms of migraine are classified as deficient *ben* 本 in combination with excessive *biao* 标. Deficient *ben* 本 is usually seen in the remission stage of migraine, in which the excessive *biao* 标 (including wind, fire, phlegm and Blood stasis) plays an important role in the acute episode. This condition mainly involves organs of the Liver, Spleen and Kidney, as well as *qi* and Blood. This chapter aims to introduce the main Chinese medicine therapies for the management of migraine, recommended by clinical guidelines, textbooks and monographs.

Introduction

In Chinese medicine (CM) theory classical literature, multiple disease names were used to describe diseases associated with headache, such as *shou feng* 首风, *nao feng* 脑风, *nao tong* 脑痛, *tou feng* 头风 and *tou tong* 头痛. Some disease names specifically refer to headache occurring on one side and have also been used in classical CM literature, including *pian tou tong* 偏头痛, *pian tou feng* 偏头风 and *pian tou teng* 偏头疼, which may be more consistent with migraine.

The disease names *shou feng* 首风 and *nao feng* 脑风 were first seen in the book *Su Wen Feng Lun* 素问·风论 around 2000 years ago, with a statement of 'when wind attacks the head from the area of *feng fu* 风府 (an acupuncture point), it results in *nao feng* 脑风; if a person is attacked by wind after hot bath, he will suffer from *shou feng* 首风. Therefore, wind attack is the main pathogenic factor which may cause many diseases' (风之所中则为偏风。风气循风府而上，则为脑风 … 新沐中风，则为首风 … 故风者，百病之长也，至其变化乃为他病，无常方，然故有风气也).

The term *tou feng* 头风 was found in the book *Zhu Bing Yuan Hou Lun* 诸病源候论•头面风候 (610 AD); it was pointed out that such condition was caused by external wind attack to *yang* meridians with underlying internal deficiency, and the main symptom (headache) may be episodic as well as last for many years (头面风者，是体虚，诸阳经脉为风所乘也，又新沐头未干，不可以卧，使头重身热，反得风，而致头风). More detailed explanation of *tou feng* 头风 was recorded in *Ren Zhai Zhi Zhi Fang* 仁斋直指方 (1264 AD), stating that '*tou feng* 头风 is not necessary to present the symptom of headache; other symptoms such as change of sensations, dizziness and yawning are often shown in the early stage of *tou feng* 头风'. This description is somehow consistent with the current understanding of migraine prodrome and aura (头风为病，不必须有偏正头疼之证，但自颈项以上，耳目口鼻眉棱之间，或有一处不若吾之体焉，皆其渐也。有头疼，有头运，有头皮顽厚).

The more specific term, *pian tou tong* 偏头痛, was first seen in the book *Ru Men Shi Qin* 儒门事亲 (1228 AD), defining that single-sided headache between frontal angle and ear is called *pian tou tong* 偏头痛 (病额角上，耳上痛，俗呼为偏头痛). Another book, *Dong Yuan Shi Shu* 东垣十书•内外伤辨 (1529 AD), also pointed out that 'single-sided headache is called *pian tou tong* 偏头痛 (如头半边痛者……此偏头痛也), and *pian zheng tou feng* 偏正头风 is usually caused by wind-cold attacking the upper part of body and remaining in *yang* 阳 meridians' (风寒伤上部，入客于经络，令人振寒头痛；或风寒之邪，伏留阳经，为偏正头风).

In the Ming dynasty, the books *Zheng Zhi Zhun Sheng* 证治准绳 (1602 AD) and *Yi Zong Bi Du* 医宗必读 (1637 AD) separated the diseases *tou tong* 头痛 and *tou feng* 头风, with *tou tong* 头痛 being an acute condition while *tou feng* 头风 was a chronic condition (经知新而暴者名头痛，深而久者名头风) (头痛头风为二门，然一病也，但有新

久去留之分耳。浅而近者名头痛，其痛卒然而至，易于解散速安
也；深而远者为头风，其痛作止不常，愈后遇触复发也).[1,2]

Aetiology and Pathogenesis

According to CM theory, migraine is commonly classified as head-ache caused by internal pathogenesis. Since all *yang* meridians travel to the head, and the Liver meridian and the Governor (GV) meridian 督脉 meet on top of the head, it is possible that headache can be caused by the pathogenesis of multiple organs or meridians. When external wind-cold or damp-heat attacks the head, or phlegm and Blood stagnate the head, the normal *qi* 气 movement will be disturbed. Abnormal *qi* uprising or blockage will cause pain. The main types of aetiology are presented below.

- **Liver *yang* uprising causing internal wind, disturbing the clear orifices.** The organ Liver stores Blood and carries functions based on *yin* and Blood. For example, if a person is born with Liver-Kidney *yin* deficiency, he or she would suffer from hyperactive Liver *yang* which may ascend to obstruct the Brain and finally result in headaches. If Liver *qi* is stagnated, it may turn into fire, which can ascend and disturb the Brain, and cause headaches.
- **Spleen dysfunction failing in transportation and transformation, causing insufficient nourishment of the Brain.** Such aetiology could be developed in two ways: (1) unhealthy diet and overworking may cause dysfunction of the Spleen; then the lack of transportation and transformation will further cause internal phlegm and dampness accumulation, blocking the channels through which the *qi* and Blood nourish the Brain and therefore cause headaches; (2) when the Spleen is not functioning, there will not be sufficient *qi* and Blood generated; therefore the Brain will not be nourished and headaches may occur.
- **Kidney deficiency.** Kidney deficiency causes headaches in two ways: (1) Kidney *yin* deficiency will cause a lack of nourishing of the Liver (not enough water to nourish wood); then Liver *yin* deficiency

will cause internal wind to disturb the clear orifices and then headaches occur; (2) the Brain is also called as 'Marrow-sea', and the Kidney is the organ producing Essence, a substance which will transfer to Marrow to fill the Brain. When the Essence is insufficient, whether congenitally or not produced sufficiently, the Brain (Marrow-sea) will not be full and therefore headaches occur.

- ***Qi* stagnation and Blood stasis.** Injuries or chronic diseases will cause *qi* stagnation and Blood stasis, blocking meridians and therefore headaches occur.

In summary, migraine is caused by multiple factors including wind, fire, phlegm, *qi* stagnation and Blood stasis, as well as the dysfunction of organs in combination of external pathogens. The symptoms of migraine are classified as deficient *ben* 本 (meaning the root, the fundamental part) in combination with excessive *biao* 标 (meaning the superficial part). Deficient *ben* 本 is usually seen in the remission stage of migraine, while the excessive *biao* 标 plays an important role in the acute episode.[3–5]

Chinese Medicine Treatments Based on Syndrome Differentiation

Being one type of headache, which is caused by internal pathogenesis, migraine is a chronic and episodic disease. The treatments for migraine are firstly divided into two stages: the episodic exacerbation stage and remission stage. In the episodic exacerbation stage, the symptoms are mainly caused by excessive pathogenesis (e.g. cold, damp-heat, Liver *yang* uprising, Liver wind, Blood stasis and phlegm). In the remission stage, internal deficiency dominates the aetiology of migraine (commonly seen *qi* and Blood deficiency and Liver and Kidney deficiency). It is worth mentioning that phlegm and Blood stasis are not only pathological products but also the fundamental causes of migraine.

Secondly, the treatments for migraine should take the location of headache into consideration. According to the meridian theory, headache that occurs at the back of the head and neck is classified as *Tai yang* 太阳 meridian's disease; headaches of the forehead area is *Yang ming* 阳明 meridian's disease; headaches on the side of the head (with or without expansion to the ear) is *Shao yang* 少阳 meridian's disease; while headaches on top of the head and affecting eyes is *Jue yin* 厥阴 meridian's disease.

When treating migraine in the episodic exacerbations stage, the treatments should target eliminating the pathogenic factors, such as warming meridians to dispel the coldness, calming the Liver and suppressing *yang*, eliminating wind and reducing phlegm, activating Blood circulation and clearing heat. While in the remission stage, treatments should focus on reinforcing *qi* and Blood and nourishing Liver and Kidney. In addition, according to the location of headache, certain CM herbs could be selected to lead the treatment to specific meridians, e.g. *chuan xiong* 川芎 can be selected for *Tai yang* 太阳 headache, *bai zhi* 白芷 for *Yang ming* 阳明 headache, *chai hu* 柴胡 for *Shao yang* 少阳 headache, and *wu zhu yu* 吴茱萸 can be used for *Jue yin* 厥阴 headache.

The syndrome differentiations and treatments in this chapter are based on the recommendations in the following guidelines, expert consensus documents, textbooks and monographs (Table 2.1).[3–13]

Table 2.1. Guidelines, Expert Consensus Documents, Textbooks and Monographs

Original Title of the Guidelines, Textbooks and Monographs (in Chinese)	English Translation of the Guidelines, Textbooks and Monographs
专科专病中医临床诊疗丛书-神经科专病中医临床诊治	Chinese Medicine Clinical Guidelines: The Diagnosis and Treatment for Neurology in Chinese Medicine
循证针灸临床实践指南	Evidence-Based Clinical Guidelines of Acupuncture
现代中医神经病学	Modern Chinese Medicine in Neurology
中医内科常见病诊疗指南 (西医疾病部分) 偏头痛	Guidelines for Diagnosis and Treatment of Internal Diseases in Chinese Medicine: Migraine

(Continued)

Table 2.1. (*Continued*)

Original Title of the Guidelines, Textbooks and Monographs (in Chinese)	English Translation of the Guidelines, Textbooks and Monographs
实用中西医结合神经病学	Practical Neurology in Integrative Medicine
中医脑病学	Chinese Medicine for Neurology
中西医结合神经病学临床新进展	The Latest Integrative Medicine for Neurology
中国药典2015版	Chinese Pharmacopoeia (2015 Edition)
实用中医脑病学	Practical Chinese Medicine in Neurology
中西医结合治疗难治神经病的良方妙法	Integrative Medicine for Refractory Conditions in Neurology
针灸脑病学	Acupuncture in Encephalopathy

Chinese Herbal Medicine

Oral Chinese Herbal Medicine Based on Syndrome Differentiation

Oral CHM are recommended to be prescribed according to patients' syndrome differentiation types. It should be pointed out that the use of some herbs/ingredients may be restricted in some countries e.g. herbs such as *xi xin* 细辛. Readers are advised to comply with relevant regulations.

Liver Yang Uprising 肝阳上亢

Symptoms: Headache with distending pain, dizziness, bitter taste in mouth and dry throat; dysphoria with feverish sensation in the chest, palms and soles; hot sensations in face; yellow urine; constipation; red tongue body with yellow tongue coating, or red tongue body with little tongue coating; and rapid and wiry pulse.[3,6–9]

Treatment principle: Calming the Liver and suppressing *yang* 平肝潜阳.

Formula: Modified *Tian ma gou teng yin* 天麻钩藤饮 (originated from *Za Bing Zheng Zhi Xin Yi* 杂病证治新义).

Herbs: *Tian ma* 天麻, *gou teng* 钩藤, *du zhong* 杜仲, *shan zhi zi* 山栀子, *huang qin* 黄芩, *niu xi* 牛膝, *shi jue ming* 石决明, *sang ji sheng* 桑寄生, *yi mu cao* 益母草, *fu shen* 茯神 and *ye jiao teng* 夜交藤.

Main action of herbs: *Tian ma* 天麻 and *gou teng* 钩藤 calm the Liver and eliminate wind; *shi jue ming* 石决明 works for calming the Liver and suppressing *yang*; *niu xi* 牛膝 leads the uprising *qi* and Blood to travel to the lower part of the body; *shan zhi zi* 山栀子 and *huang qin* 黄芩 function to clear heat; *fu shen* 茯神 and *ye jiao teng* 夜交藤 are helpful in calming the mind; *yi mu cao* 益母草 can eliminate wind by nourishing Blood; *sang ji sheng* 桑寄生 and *du zhong* 杜仲 may expel wind by tonifying the Liver and Kidney.

Phlegm Stagnation in the Orifices 痰浊蒙窍

Symptoms: Headache and dizziness, fullness of the chest and epigastrium, nausea, tiredness of the body, heaviness of the limbs, poor appetite, enlarged tongue body with teeth marks, white greasy tongue coating, deep and wiry pulse, or deep and slippery pulse.[3,6–9]

Treatment principle: Fortifying the Spleen and eliminating phlegm; opening the orifices to relieve pain 健脾化痰, 通窍止痛.

Formula: Modified *Ban xia bai zhu tian ma tang* 半夏白术天麻汤 (originated from *Yi Xue Xin Wu* 医学心悟).

Herbs: *Fa ban xia* 法半夏, *bai zhu* 白术, *tian ma* 天麻, *chen pi* 陈皮, *fu ling* 茯苓, *tian nan xing* 天南星, *zhi shi* 枳实, *chuan xiong* 川芎, *bai zhi* 白芷, *cang zhu* 苍术, *ci ji li* 刺蒺藜 and *jiang can* 僵蚕.

Main action of herbs: *Tian ma* 天麻 eliminates wind; *chen pi* 陈皮, *tian nan xing* 天南星, *cang zhu* 苍术, *fa ban xia* 法半夏 and *zhi shi* 枳实 reduce dampness and phlegm; *bai zhu* 白术 and *fu ling* 茯苓 function together to tonify the Spleen and dispel dampness; *bai zhi* 白芷 opens the orifices to relieve pain; *chuan xiong* 川芎 works to remove Blood stasis to relieve pain; *ci ji li* 刺蒺藜 and *jiang can* 僵蚕 eliminate wind and smooth meridians to relieve pain.

Blood Stasis in Orifices 瘀血阻窍

Symptoms: Chronic severe headache (piercing or stabbing pain) with fixed location, may have a history of head injury; dark facial complexion; purple lips, purple tongue body with dark marks or spots; thin white tongue coating; deep and thready pulse or thready and unsmooth pulse.[3,6–9]

Treating principle: Activating Blood and removing stasis to relieve pain 活血祛瘀, 通窍止痛.

Formula: *Tong qiao huo xue tang* 通窍活血汤 (originated from *Yi Lin Gai Cuo* 医林改错).

Herbs: *Chuan xiong* 川芎, *chi shao* 赤芍, *tao ren* 桃仁, *hong hua* 红花, *dan shen* 丹参, *bai zhi* 白芷, *chai hu* 柴胡, *yan hu suo* 延胡索, *yu jin* 郁金 and *shi chang pu* 石菖蒲.

Main action of herbs: *Chuan xiong* 川芎, *chi shao* 赤芍, *tao ren* 桃仁, *hong hua* 红花 and *dan shen* 丹参 all work by activating Blood and removing Blood stasis to relieve pain; *bai zhi* 白芷 opens the orifices to relieve pain; *chai hu* 柴胡 moves *qi* to help activate Blood; while *yan hu suo* 延胡索 and *yu jin* 郁金 move *qi* and activate Blood at the same time; and *shi chang pu* 石菖蒲 removes phlegm to open the orifices.

Qi and Blood Deficiency 气血亏虚

Symptoms: Chronic ongoing mild headache, may be aggravated due to over-working, weak body and spirit, tastelessness, pale facial complexion, pale tongue body with white coating, and deep, weak, thready pulse.[3,6,8,9]

Treating principle: Tonifying *qi* and Blood, dispelling wind to relieve pain 益气补血, 祛风止痛.

Formula: Modified *Ba zhen tang* 八珍汤 (originated from *Rui Zhu Tang Jing Yan Fang* 瑞竹堂经验方).

Herbs: *Dang gui* 当归, *shu di huang* 熟地黄, *bai shao* 白芍, *chuan xiong* 川芎, *dang shen* 党参, *bai zhu* 白术, *huang qi* 黄芪, *ci ji li*

刺蒺藜, *bai zhi* 白芷, *fa ban xia* 法半夏, *sheng ma* 升麻 and *gan cao* 甘草.

Main action of herbs: *Dang gui* 当归, *shu di huang* 熟地黄, *bai shao* 白芍 and *chuan xiong* 川芎 function to tonify Blood; *dang shen* 党参, *bai zhu* 白术 and *huang qi* 黄芪 specialise in fortifying the Spleen and replenishing *qi*; *ci ji li* 刺蒺藜 expels wind and relieves pain; *bai zhi* 白芷 opens the orifices and eases pain; *fa ban xia* 法半夏 tonifies the Spleen and reduces phlegm; and *sheng ma* 升麻 ascends the clear *qi* 气 to the head and relieves pain.

Liver and Kidney Yin Deficiency 肝肾阴虚

Symptoms: Headache and dizziness, blurred vision, soreness and weakness of waist and knees, weak body and spirit, tinnitus, insomnia, feverish sensation in chest, palms and soles, red tongue body with little coating, and weak, thready pulse.[3,6,8,9]

Treating principle: Tonifying the Liver and Kidney 补益肝肾.

Formula: *Qi ju di huang wan* 杞菊地黄丸 (originated from *Ma Zhen Quan Shu* 麻疹全书)

Herbs: *Sheng di huang* 生地黄, *shan zhu yu* 山茱萸, *shan yao* 山药, *fu ling* 茯苓, *mu dan pi* 牡丹皮, *ze xie* 泽泻, *dang gui* 当归, *bai shao* 白芍, *gou qi zi* 枸杞子, *ju hua* 菊花 and *tian ma* 天麻.

Main action of herbs: *Sheng di huang* 生地黄 and *shan zhu yu* 山茱萸 function to tonify the Liver and Kidney; *shan yao* 山药 and *fu ling* 茯苓 work to tonify the Spleen; *mu dan pi* 牡丹皮 and *ze xie* 泽泻 reduce deficient heat; *bai shao* 白芍, *gou qi zi* 枸杞子 and *ju hua* 菊花 clear the Liver and improve eyesight; *dang gui* 当归 tonifies Blood and *yin* 阴; and *tian ma* 天麻 relieves pain.

Cold Stagnated in the Liver Meridian 寒凝肝脉

Symptoms: Severe pulling pain, often occurring on the top of the head; dark (blue) facial complexion; nausea and water-like vomit;

sometimes with cold extremities and purple lips; pale or purple tongue body, with thin and white coating; and deep and thready pulse.[6,8]

Treating principle: Warming the meridian, dispelling coldness, activating the Blood and unblocking meridians 温经散寒, 活血通络.

Formula: *Wu zhu yu tang* 吴茱萸汤 (originated from *Shang Han Lun* 伤寒论).

Herbs: *Wu zhu yu* 吴茱萸, *sheng jiang* 生姜, *chuan xiong* 川芎, *bai zhi* 白芷, *gao ben* 藁本 and *gan cao* 甘草.

Main action of herbs: *Wu zhu yu* 吴茱萸 functions to warm the Liver meridian and dispel coldness; *sheng jiang* 生姜 warms the body; *chuan xiong* 川芎 warms the meridians and activates Blood; *bai zhi* 白芷 and *gao ben* 藁本 help to dispel coldness and relieve pain; and *gan cao* 甘草 harmonises all herbs of a formula.

Commonly Used Chinese Herbal Medicine Commercial Products

Tong Tian Kou Fu Ye 通天口服液

Herbs: *Chuan xiong* 川芎, *chi shao* 赤芍, *tian ma* 天麻, *qiang huo* 羌活, *bai zhi* 白芷, *xi xin* 细辛, *ju hua* 菊花, *bo he* 薄荷, *fang feng* 防风, *cha ye* 茶叶 and *gan cao* 甘草.

Function: Activating Blood circulation and removing Blood stasis, dispelling wind and relieving pain. This medication is suitable for migraine caused by Blood stasis and wind attacking.

Dosage: Oral — taking one dose each time, three times a day, three days for a course of treatment.[3,6,7,10]

Quan Tian Ma Jiao Nang 全天麻胶囊

Herbs: *Tian ma* 天麻.

Function: Calming the Liver and expelling wind. This is suitable for headache caused by Liver wind uprising.

Dosage: Oral — taking two to six capsules each time, three times a day, 15 days for a course of treatment.[3,6,8,10]

Zheng Tian Wan 正天丸

Herbs: *Gou teng* 钩藤, *bai shao* 白芍, *chuan xiong* 川芎, *dang gui* 当归, *di huang* 地黄, *bai zhi* 白芷, *fang feng* 防风, *qiang huo* 羌活, *tao ren* 桃仁, *hong hua* 红花, *xi xin* 细辛, *du huo* 独活, *ma huang* 麻黄, *fu zi* 附子 and *ji xue teng* 鸡血藤.

Function: Dispelling wind and activating Blood circulation, soothing the Liver and tonifying the Blood, unblocking meridians and relieving pain. This is suitable for migraine caused by external wind attacking, Blood stasis, Blood deficiency and Liver *yang* uprising.

Dosage: Oral — taking six grams each time after meals, two or three times per day, 15 days for a course of treatment.[5,10]

Fu Fang Yang Jiao Pian 复方羊角片 *or* *Fu Fang Yang Jiao Ke Li* 复方羊角颗粒

Herbs: *Shan yang jiao* 山羊角, *chuan xiong* 川芎, *bai zhi* 白芷 and *zhi chuan wu* 制川乌.

Function: Soothing the Liver and dispelling wind, unblocking meridians to relieve pain. This is suitable for migraine caused by Liver wind and Blood stasis.

Dosage: Oral — taking five pills each time, three times a day.[6,10]

Xue Fu Zhu Yu Kou Fu Ye 血府逐瘀口服液 *or Xue Fu Zhu Yu Jiao Nang* 血府逐瘀胶囊

Herbs: *Chai hu* 柴胡, *dang gui* 当归, *di huang* 地黄, *chi shao* 赤芍, *hong hua* 红花, *tao ren* 桃仁, *zhi ke* 枳壳, *gan cao* 甘草, *chuan xiong* 川芎, *niu xi* 牛膝 and *jie geng* 桔梗.

Function: Activating Blood circulation, moving *qi* to relieve pain. This is suitable for headache caused by *qi* stagnation and Blood stasis.

Dosage: Oral solution — taking 20 ml each time, three times a day; capsule — one or two capsules each time, twice a day.[6,7,8,10]

Yang Xue Qing Nao Ke Li 养血清脑颗粒

Herbs: *Dang gui* 当归, *chuan xiong* 川芎, *bai shao* 白芍, *shu di huang* 熟地黄, *gou teng* 钩藤, *xia ku cao* 夏枯草, *ji xue teng* 鸡血藤, *jue ming zi* 决明子, *zhen zhu mu* 珍珠母, *yan hu suo* 延胡索 and *xi xin* 细辛.

Function: Soothing the Liver and nourishing Blood, activating Blood circulation. This is suitable for headache caused by Blood deficiency with Liver hyperactivity.

Dosage: Oral — taking one package (3 g) each time, three times a day.[6,8,10]

Tian Ma Tou Tong Pian 天麻头痛片

Herbs: *Tian ma* 天麻, *bai zhi* 白芷, *chuan xiong* 川芎, *jing jie* 荆芥, *dang gui* 当归 and *ru xiang* 乳香.

Function: Nourishing Blood and dispelling wind, removing coldness to relieve pain. This is suitable for migraine caused by Blood deficiency and Blood stasis.

Dosage: Oral — taking four to six tablets each time, three times a day.[6,10]

Chinese Herbal Medicine Sniffing

Grind together one centipede and *bing pian* 冰片 (0.6 g) to a powder; sniff the powder to trigger sneezing. This is suitable for migraine acute stage (Blood stasis type). One sniff in every three hours.[8]

Chinese Herbal Medicine External Application

Herbs: *Di long* 地龙, *quan xie* 全蝎, *lu lu tong* 路路通, *sheng nan xing* 生南星, *sheng bai xia* 生半夏, *bai fu zi* 白附子 and *xi xin* 细辛.

Method: Mix all the above herbs and grind them to a powder, then add starch to make a paste. Apply the paste on the area of EX-HN5

Taiyang 太阳, once a day. This therapy is suitable for headaches caused by Blood stasis in orifices.[8]

Chinese Herbal Medicine Fumigation and Steaming Therapy

Herbs: *Xi xin* 细辛, *shi chang pu* 石菖蒲, *qiang huo* 羌活, *zi su ye* 紫苏叶, *chuan xiong* 川芎 and *jiang can* 僵蚕.

Method: Mix the above-listed herbs in a pot, and bring the mixture to a boil. Then apply steaming therapy using the decoction. This method is suitable for migraine caused by phlegm stagnation in orifices.[8]

Acupuncture Therapy

Treating principle: Moving *qi* and activating Blood, unblocking the *Shao yang* 少阳 meridian.

Treatment plan should differ for the different stages of migraine: (1) in the acute stage of migraine, points should be selected from *Shao yang* 少阳 meridian points or local *Ashi* points 阿是穴; (2) in the remission stage of migraine, points should be selected according to syndrome differentiation.[4]

Acupuncture techniques including body acupuncture, scalp acupuncture, ear acupuncture or acupressure, and moxibustion can be selected.

Body Acupuncture (Electroacupuncture)

Body acupuncture is frequently used in clinical practice for the management of migraine. The below recommended acupuncture points and methods are summarised from clinical guidelines, textbooks and monographs.[4,6,7,8,13]

Acute Stage

In the acute stage of migraine, acupuncture therapy is mainly applied on local *Ashi* points or points from *Shao yang* 少阳 meridians, as described below.

Main points: *Ashi* points, TE23 *Sizhukong* 丝竹空, GB8 *Shuaigu* 率谷, EX-HN5 *Taiyang* 太阳, GB20 *Fengchi* 风池, LI4 *Hegu* 合谷, LR3 *Taichong* 太冲 and GB41 *Zulinqi* 足临泣.

Additional points: GB34 *Yanglingquan* 阳陵泉 and TE5 *Waiguan* 外关.

Method: Select relevant points (local points unilateral, distal points bilateral); point-to-point needling can be used for TE23 *Sizhukong* 丝竹空 and GB8 *Shuaigu* 率谷; electroacupuncture can be used for *Ashi* points, 30 minutes for each session, 10 sessions (once in every two days) as a treatment course.

Remission Stage

In addition to the local points and *Shao yang* 少阳 meridian points, other points can also be selected for acupuncture (or electroacupuncture) for the remission stage of migraine, as described below:

- Liver yang uprising: From GB4 *Hanyan* 颔厌 to GB5 *Xuanlu* 悬颅, LU7 *Lieque* 列缺, KI3 *Taixi* 太溪 and LR2 *Xingjian* 行间;
- Phlegm stagnation: From GB4 *Hanyan* 颔厌 to GB5 *Xuanlu* 悬颅, LU7 *Lieque* 列缺, ST40 *Fenglong* 丰隆 and PC6 *Neiguan* 内关;
- Blood stasis: BL17 *Geshu* 膈俞, SP10 *Xuehai* 血海, ST36 *Zusanli* 足三里 and SP6 *Sanyinjiao* 三阴交;
- Kidney, *qi* and Blood deficiency: ST36 *Zusanli* 足三里, CV6 *Qihai* 气海, SP6 *Sanyinjiao* 三阴交, KI3 *Taixi* 太溪 and BL23 *Shenshu* 肾俞.

Method: Selecting relevant points, apply acupuncture for 30 minutes in each session, one session in every two days, ten sessions as a treatment course. Electroacupuncture can also be applied.

Scalp Acupuncture 头皮针

Scalp acupuncture is usually used for the acute stage.[3,4]

Main points: MS7, posterior oblique line of vertex-temporal on the opposite side; MS8 and MS9, lateral line one and two of vertex.

Additional points: With pain in fronto-temporal area, add GB8 *Shuaigu* 率谷; with pain in the top of head, add GB20 *Fengchi* 风池; with symptoms of *Jueyin* 厥阴 meridian, add PC6 *Neiguan* 内关, GV26 *Shuigou* 水沟, HT7 *Shenmen* 神门 and GV20 *Baihui* 百会; with symptoms of *Yangming* 阳明 meridian, add ST8 *Touwei* 头维; and with symptoms of Bladder meridian, add BL10 *Tianzhu* 天柱.

Method: Selecting relevant points, electroacupuncture can be applied in addition to acupuncture. Needles on scalp points can be retained for 60 minutes; needles on other body points will be retained for 30 minutes; one session in every two days, ten sessions as a treatment course.

Ear Acupuncture and Ear Acupressure

Ear acupuncture using specially designed needles or ear acupressure using pellets are options for migraine management.[3,4,6,7,11–13]

Points: TF4 *Shenmen* 神门, AT4 Subcortex 皮质下, AT3 Occiput 枕 and AT1 Forehead 额.

Method: Needle at two or three points as above, retaining for 20–30 minutes, or use pressing pellets for ear acupressure on the above points.

Moxibustion

Points: EX-HN5 *Taiyang* 太阳, GB20 *Fengchi* 风池, GV20 *Baihui* 百会, GB8 *Shuaigu* 率谷, GB22 *Xinhui* 囟会, EX-HN3 *Yintang* 印堂, LR2 *Xingjian* 行间, BL10 *Tianzhu* 天柱 and TE5 *Waiguan* 外关.

Method: Applying stick moxibustion on the above points, select two to four points each time, five to ten minutes for each point, one to two sessions each day. This method is suitable for migraine caused by *qi* and Blood deficiency or Kidney deficiency.[13]

Tuina 推拿 **Therapy**

Tuina 推拿 therapy can be used for relieving migraine symptoms. Local acupuncture points could be selected for *tuina* 推拿 therapy in combination with distal points according to syndrome differentiation.[6]

Points: Local points including EX-HN3 *Yintang* 印堂, EX-HN5 *Taiyang* 太阳, GV20 *Baihui* 百会, GB20 *Fengchi* 风池, BL1 *Jingming* 睛明 and ST8 *Touwe* 头维穴. Distal points including LI4 *Hegu* 合谷, LI11 *Quchi* 曲池, ST36 *Zusanli* 足三里 and LR2 *Xingjian* 行间. *Tuina* 推拿 therapy should be applied on both local points and distal points. This is suitable for acute stage of migraine.

Method: Common *tuina* 推拿 therapy methods are *qi*-concentrated single-finger manipulation 指禅推法, grasping manipulation 拿法, pressing 按法, kneading manipulation 揉法, rolling 𢷼法, etc.

In addition to the above listed points, other points can be selected according to syndrome differentiation as described below.

- Cold stagnated in the Liver meridian: Press and knead the points of GV20 *Baihui* 百会, ST36 *Zusanli* 足三里 and KI1 *Yongquan* 涌泉.
- Liver *yang* 阳 uprising: Push *qiaogong* 桥弓, which is located on the sides of the neck (sternocleidomastoid) for 20 times one side after another, then knead and press LR3 *Taichong* 太冲 and LR2 *Xingjian* 行间, and scrub KI1 *Yongquan* 涌泉.
- Phlegm and wind uprising: Apply *qi*-concentrated single-finger manipulation 指禅推法 and rubbing manipulation 摩法 on the abdomen, focusing on CV12 *Zhongwan* 中脘 and ST25 *Tianshu* 天枢 for three minutes; then apply pressing 按法 and kneading manipulation 揉法 on BL20 *Pishu* 脾俞, BL21 *Weishu* 胃俞, ST36 *Zusanli* 足三里 and ST40 *Fenglong* 丰隆 for three minutes.
- Blood stasis in meridians: Apply kneading manipulation 揉法 and *qi*-concentrated single-finger manipulation 指禅推法 on the *Ashi* points for five minutes, then scrub the forehead and EX-HN5 *Taiyang* 太阳 after applying some Holly ointment 冬青膏 on the skin until feeling hot in these areas. Finally, apply pressing 按法

and kneading manipulation 揉法 on BL17 *Geshu* 膈俞, SP10 *Xuehai* 血海 and SP6 *Sanyinjiao* 三阴交 for five minutes.

Lifestyle Adjustment and Avoiding Triggers

Diet control: Avoid food which may induce headache, including alcohol.[7]

Lifestyle: Avoid cold, lack of sleep or mood swing.[4]

Prognosis

Migraine is believed to be incurable, but with proper management and as they age, migraineurs may gradually achieve pain relief and reduction in migraine frequency.[9,14]

Table 2.2 is a brief summary of recommended Chinese medicine therapies for migraine.

Table 2.2. Summary of Chinese Medicine Treatments

Types of Chinese Herbal Medicine	Chinese Herbal Medicine Treatment	
	Syndromes	**Formula**
Oral Chinese herbal medicine	Liver *yang* uprising 肝阳上亢	Modified *Tian ma gou teng yin* 天麻钩藤饮
	Phlegm stagnation in the orifices 痰浊蒙窍	Modified *Ban xia bai zhu tian ma tang* 半夏白术天麻汤
	Blood stasis in orifices 瘀血阻窍	*Tong qiao huo xue tang* 通窍活血汤
	Qi and Blood deficiency 气血亏虚	Modified *Ba zhen tang* 八珍汤
	Liver and Kidney *yin* deficiency 肝肾阴虚	*Qi ju di huang wan* 杞菊地黄丸
	Cold stagnated in the Liver meridian 寒凝肝脉	*Wu zhu yu tang* 吴茱萸汤

(Continued)

Table 2.2.   (*Continued*)

Types of Chinese Herbal Medicine	Chinese Herbal Medicine Treatment	
	Syndromes	**Formula**
	Tong tian kou fu ye 通天口服液	
	Quan tian ma jiao nang 全天麻胶囊	
	Zheng tian wan 正天丸	
	Fu fang yang jiao pian 复方羊角片, *Fu fang yang jiao ke li* 复方羊角颗粒	
	Xue fu zhu yu kou fu ye 血府逐瘀口服液, *Xue fu zhu yu jiao nang* 血府逐瘀胶囊	
	Yang xue qing nao ke li 养血清脑颗粒	
	Tian ma tou tong pian 天麻头痛片	
Topical Chinese herbal medicine	Chinese herbal medicine sniffing	
	Chinese herbal medicine external application	
	Chinese herbal medicine fumigation and steaming therapy	
Acupuncture Therapies		
Body acupuncture	Acute stage	On local *Ashi* points or points from *Shaoyang* 少阳 meridians.
	Remission stage	Select acupuncture points according to syndrome differentiation.
Scalp acupuncture	Scalp acupuncture is usually used for acute stage.	
Ear acupuncture and ear acupressure	Needle at two or three points, retaining for 20–30 minutes, or use pressing pellets for ear acupressure on the above points.	
Moxibustion	This method is suitable for migraine caused by *qi* and Blood deficiency or Kidney deficiency.	
***Tuina* 推拿 Therapy**		
Tuina 推拿 therapy can be applied on local points and additional distal points according to syndrome differentiation.		

References

1. 吴玉斌. (2014) 论'头风'病源流. 辽宁中医药大学学报 **16(01):** 136–137.
2. 黎婉玲. (2012) 偏头痛患者的中医体质特征研究 (Thesis). 南方医科大学.
3. 黄培新, 黄燕. (2013) 专科专病中医临床诊疗丛书●神经科专病中医临床诊治. 北京: 人民卫生出版社.
4. 中国针灸学会. (2014) 循证针灸临床实践指南. 北京: 中国中医药出版社.
5. 鲍远程. (2003) 现代中医神经病学. 北京: 人民卫生出版社.
6. 曹克刚, 高颖. (2011) 中医内科常见病诊疗指南 (西医疾病部分) 偏头痛. 中国中医药现代远程教育. 北京: 中国中医药出版社. 275–278.
7. 孙怡. (2011) 实用中西医结合神经病学. 北京: 人民卫生出版社.
8. 王永炎, 张伯礼. (2007) 中医脑病学. 北京: 人民卫生出版社.
9. 胡学强. (2015) 中西医结合神经病学临床新进展. 北京: 人民军医出版社.
10. 国家药典委员会. (2015) 中华人民共和国药典. 北京: 中国医药科技出版社.
11. 阎孝诚. (1993) 实用中医脑病学. 北京: 学苑出版社.
12. 吴大真. (2001) 中西医结合治疗难治神经病的良方妙法. 北京: 中国医药科技出版社.
13. 赖新生. (2006) 针灸脑病学. 北京: 人民卫生出版社.
14. 梁繁荣. (2016) 针灸学. 北京: 中国中医出版社.

3

Classical Chinese Medicine Literature

OVERVIEW

Classical Chinese medicine literature provides a rich source of information for the prevention and management of disease. There may be some treatments used in contemporary practice that date back to classical literature, including current treatments for migraine. This chapter describes the findings of a systematic search of the *Zhong Hua Yi Dian* 中华医典, based on a selection of search terms identified from classical dictionaries and texts. A total of 1,856 citations were analysed to identify the common formulas, herbs and acupuncture points used to treat symptoms 'possibly' or 'likely' corresponding to migraine.

Introduction

Chinese medicine (CM) therapies have been practised for thousands of years. For example, acupuncture is commonly thought to originate in ancient China 2,500 years ago during the late Spring and Autumn (770–476 BC) or early Warring States (474–221 BC) periods,[1,2] and the book *Shen Nong Ben Cao Jing* 神农本草经 [*Shennong's Materia Medica*], is generally believed to be the oldest surviving book on materia medica presenting the earliest practice of Chinese herbal medicine (CHM) in the Western Han dynasty (206 BC–24 AD).[3,4]

During the thousands of years of CM clinical practice, a large amount of literature has accumulated, recording the aetiology and treatments for clinical conditions including different types of headache. Migraine was considered as one type of headache with specific clinical features and syndrome differentiation (see Chapter 2). The treatments for migraine using CHM or acupuncture-related therapies may also have been recorded in the vast classical literature. However, to comprehensively locate all CM treatments for migraine from classical literature is challenging, since migraine was not clearly defined as a specific disease in history. In order to systematically summarise such information from the vast classical CM literature, the digitalised collections *Zhong Hua Yi Dian* (ZHYD) 中华医典 CD-ROM (a collection of more than 1,000 medical books of the classical CM literature) was accessed. This collection is the largest currently available and is representative of other large collections of the classical and pre-modern CM literature.[3–5]

Search Terms

The disease name 'migraine' in Chinese language is *pian tou tong* 偏头痛, which refers to 'headache on one side of the head', describing the main feature of this condition. Since it is not necessary that migraine only occurs as headache on one side of the head, and there are up to 40% of cases that suffer pain on both sides of the head during migraine attacks,[6] in order to summarise all possible treatments for migraine as comprehensively as possible, it is important to investigate all types of headaches recorded in classical literature. Therefore, we firstly examined previously published monographs,[7–10] clinical guidelines,[11,12] journal articles and theses[13–21] which explained the terminology and aetiology of migraine in the CM concept, selected possible terms which were then discussed with clinical experts, and lastly identified a total of 22 terms to be used for searching ZHYD for potential treatments for adult migraine (Table 3.1).

Procedures for Searches, Data Coding and Data Analysis

Each term was entered into the ZHYD search fields and the search results were downloaded to spreadsheets. Duplicate results caused by different search terms were removed. A 'citation' was defined as a

Table 3.1. Terms Used to Identify Classical Literature Citations

Search Terms of Migraine in Pinyin	Search Terms of Migraine in Chinese	English Translation
Shou feng	首风	Wind invasion on the head
Nao feng	脑风	Wind invasion on the head
Tou teng	头疼	Headache
Pian tou teng	偏头疼	Headache on one side of the head
Pian zheng tou teng	偏正头疼	Headache on one side and the middle of the head
Tou tong	头痛	Headache
Pian tou tong	偏头痛	Headache on one side of the head
Ban bian tou tong	半边头痛	Headache on one side of the head
Pian zheng tou tong	偏正头痛	Headache on one side and the middle of the head
Jue tou tong	厥头痛	Headache caused by pathogeneses rising
Tou feng	头风	Wind invasion on the head
Pian zheng tou feng	偏正头风	Wind invasion on one side and the middle of the head
Pian tou feng	偏头风	Wind invasion on one side of the head
Ban bian tou feng	半边头风	Wind invasion on one side of the head
Tou feng pian tong	头风偏痛	Wind invasion and pain on one side of the head
Nao tong	脑痛	Headache
Pian nao tong	偏脑痛	Headache on one side of the head
Tou pian tong	头偏痛	Headache on one side of the head
Pian tou huan	偏头患	Disease on one side of the head
Tou ban bian tong	头半边痛	Headache on one side of the head
Tou ban han tong	头半寒痛	Headache and coldness on one side of the head
Tou xiang pian tong	头项偏痛	Headache and neck pain on one side of the head and neck

distinct passage of text referring to one or more of the search terms. Citations were excluded from further analyses if they described treatments targeting children, or secondary headaches caused by other reasons including wind-cold invasion, brain tumour, pestilence or infectious disease, malaria, alcohol intake and syphilis. Some citations may have described symptoms of primary headache but are more likely to refer to cluster headache or prosopalgia; these citations were also excluded through discussion. It should be pointed out that some citations described typical migraine symptoms (e.g. one-sided headache accompanied with nausea, vomiting and photophobia), but there were other symptoms unlikely to be migraine such as severe eye pain; these citations were judged as more likely to be glaucoma and therefore they were also excluded. Furthermore, some citations that contain the disease name *tou feng* 头风 but referred to other external conditions (e.g. accompanied with itch and dandruff) rather than headache, were excluded. Some citations described other types of headache, for example, headaches caused by glaucoma (accompanied with eye symptoms), trigeminal neuralgia and cluster headache. These were also excluded.

All relevant citations were reviewed to identify the best descriptions of migraine and its aetiology or pathogenesis. Relevant citations which did not include treatment were excluded from further analyses. Citations which were pharmacopeia-type entries were reviewed for eligibility. Pharmacopeia entries which mentioned the name of the condition but did not include a detailed description of the condition or information about treatment were excluded from further analysis. Pharmacopeia entries which included a description of the condition, with or without reference to other herbs, were included. Citations that introduced acupuncture points' targeting diseases and treatment methods of using those points were included. Since migraine is often treated by acupuncture-related therapies applied on certain meridians corresponding to the location of pain, those citations that introduced meridian treatments, with or without the names of actual points, were also included for further analyses.

After exclusions, the final dataset was limited to the citations considered potentially referring to migraine with description of CM treatments (CHM, acupuncture and related therapies, or other CM therapies). Included citations were grouped according to the CM intervention for further analysis. When a citation referred to multiple treatments, each treatment was considered as a separate citation for calculation of formulas, herbs or acupuncture points.

All the relevant citations containing treatments were considered as 'possible' migraine citations. Furthermore, an additional screening process was performed to identify citations considered specifically related to migraine, which were considered as 'most likely' migraine citations. In this screening process, certain specific symptoms or disease names were scored following the methods shown in Table 3.2. The information of symptom and disease name contained in a citation

Table 3.2. Symptoms Scoring Criteria

Symptoms	Terms Referring to the Symptom	Score
Symptoms repeatedly occur	*Fu fa* 复发, *shi fa shi zhi* 时发时止, *zuo zhi bu chang* 作止不常, *zha chai zha fa* 乍差乍发 and *ta xie bu ding* 发歇不定.	1
Chronic disease	*Shen jiu* 深久, *yuan nian* 远年, *nian shen* 年深, *shu sui bu yi* 数岁已, *jiu bu yi* 久不已, *jiu bu chai* 久不瘥, *jiu bu yu* 久不愈 and *shu nian* 数年.	1
One side of the head	*Tou jiao* 头角, *ejiao* 额角 (corner of the forehead), *ban bian* 半边, *ban pan* 半爿, *yu wei* 鱼尾, *zuo* 左, *you* 右, *tai yang xue tong* 太阳穴痛 (pain in the temple region), *pian* 偏, *tou ban* 头半 and *tan yang tong* 太阳痛 (pain in the temple region).	2
Pulsing pain	*Tou zhan* 头胀 (distending pain) and *tiao tong* 跳痛 (pulsing pain).	1
Mild to severe pain	*Bu ke ren* 不可忍 and *ju tong* 剧痛.	1
Nausea and vomiting	*E xin* 恶心/*Ou* 呕.	1
Sensitivity to light and sounds	*Bu gan jian guang* 不敢见光/*Wu wen ren sheng* 恶闻人声.	1
Disease Names	**Terms Referring to the Disease Name**	
	Nao feng 脑风, *shou feng* 首风, *tou feng* 头风, *tou tong* 头痛, *tou teng* 头疼, *nao tong* 脑痛 and *jue tou tong* 厥头痛.	1

were extracted and scored; citations with a total score of greater than three were further selected as the 'most likely' migraine citations.

Search Results

The search procedure is shown in Fig. 3.1.

A total of 24,194 hits (instances of the term) were identified through heading/body text search in ZHYD by 23 search terms (Table 3.3). The terms *tou tong* 头痛 and *tou teng* 头疼, which have the same meaning of 'headache' in the Chinese language, produced the greatest number of hits with 15,713 and 4,583 hits, respectively.

Citations Related to Migraine

After duplicate removal and exclusions for all the reasons as above-mentioned, a total of 1,856 citations related to migraine met the inclusion criteria and were included for further analyses. These were considered as 'possible' migraine citations. Of these, 1,514 citations described CHM treatments in text, while 312 citations stated acupuncture-related therapies. *Daoyin* 导引 exercise, a type of *qigong* 气功 therapy, was mentioned in 19 citations. There were 11 citations

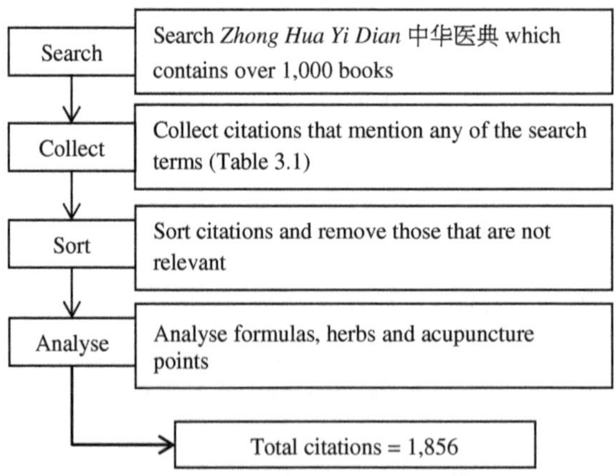

Fig. 3.1. Classical literature citations

Table 3.3. Hit Frequency by Search Term

Pinyin	Chinese Characters	Total Hit Frequency (*n,* %)
Tou tong	头痛	15,713 (64.9)
Tou teng	头疼	4,583 (18.9)
Tou feng	头风	2,313 (9.6)
Nao tong	脑痛	365 (1.5)
Pian zheng tou feng	偏正头风	223 (0.9)
Jue tou tong	厥头痛	216 (0.9)
Nao feng	脑风	212 (0.9)
Pian tou tong	偏头痛	170 (0.7)
Pian tou feng	偏头风	105 (0.4)
Pian zheng tou tong	偏正头痛	88 (0.4)
Shou feng	首风	63 (0.3)
Pian zheng tou teng	偏正头疼	38 (0.2)
Tou pian tong	头偏痛	32 (0.1)
Pian tou teng	偏头疼	29 (0.1)
Tou ban han tong	头半寒痛	19 (0.1)
Pian tou han	偏头患	9 (0.04)
Tou xiang pian tong	头项偏痛	5 (0.02)
Ban bian tou tong	半边头痛	3 (0.01)
Tou ban bian tong	头半边痛	3 (0.01)
Ban bian tou feng	半边头风	2 (0.01)
Pian nao tong	偏脑痛	1 (0.004)
Tou feng pian tong	头风偏痛	1 (0.004)

which introduced CM therapies that are not commonly used in current practice outside China; these were not included in our analyses.

All included citations were also reviewed to identify and synthesise the aetiological or pathogenic details of the disease. Non-treatment citations which described the aetiological or pathogenic details were also reviewed to identify appropriate explanations in this aspect.

By placing the criterion of 'total score greater than three', 186 citations were identified as 'most likely' migraine citations. Among these, 112 citations introduced oral CHM treatments, 64 citations included topical CHM treatments and two citations mentioned CHM treatments used both orally and topically. Ten citations included acupuncture treatment.

Definitions of the Condition and Aetiology

In history, migraine used to be described under the diseases named *tou tong* 头痛, *tou feng* 头风, *shou feng* 首风, *nao feng* 脑风, *nao tong* 脑痛, etc. Later, a specific description meaning 'one-sided' was added to these disease names; therefore terms such as *pian tou tong* 偏头痛, *pian zheng tou tong* 偏正头痛, *pian tou teng* 偏头疼, *pian zheng tou teng* 偏正头疼, *pian tou feng* 偏头风, *pian zheng tou feng* 偏正头风, *ban bian tou feng* 半边头风 and *jia nao feng* 夹脑风 started to be used.

The earliest discussion of *shou feng* 首风 and *nao feng* 脑风 was seen in *Su Wen* 素问•风论, which described that external wind attack could cause problems of the head such as headache, and these conditions may recur frequently, which is similar as wind. In the book *Zhu Bing Yuan Hou Lun* 诸病源候论•头面风候 (610 AD), it was pointed out that the occurrence of *tou mian feng* 头面风 was caused by wind attacking *yang* meridians when the body's vital energy is deficient. This is the first appearance of the term *tou feng* 头风.

In the Song dynasty (961–1271 AD) the disease *tou feng* 头风 was recorded in the book Ren Zhai Zhi Zhi Fang Lun 仁斋直指方论 (1264 AD) with more details, pointing out the specific location of the pain and its accompanying symptoms such as change of sensations, sweating and frequent yawning; some of these symptoms seem similar to the migraine aura or prodrome symptoms.

The disease name *pian tou tong* 偏头痛, which is used in current clinical practice referring to migraine, was first shown in the book *Dong Yuan Shi Shu* 东垣十书 (1529 AD). In the Ming dynasty (1369–1644 AD) clinicians differentiated migraine from common headache as migraine being a chronic recurrent condition. Examples can be found in the books *Yi Zong Bi Du* 医宗必读 (1637 AD) and *Zheng Zhi Zhun Sheng* 证治准绳 (1602 AD).

It is clear that the definitions of migraine have developed and been modified over a long period in history. Accordingly, the aetiology of migraine has also evolved. For example, it was recorded in *Nan Jing* 难经 that *jue tou tong* 厥头痛 was caused by wind cold invading the three *yang* meridians. The pain on top of the head was caused by 'stagnated *qi* not travelling up and down', as stated in *Su Wen* 素问•方盛衰论. In the Jin 晋 dynasty (266–420 AD) it was recorded that headache was often caused by *qi* uprising in the Liver and Kidney meridians in the book *Mai Jing* 脉经•头痛 (258 AD). In the Yuan dynasty (1272–1368 AD), *Dan Xi Xin Fa* 丹溪心法•头痛 (1347 AD) stated that the disease *tou feng* 头风 was caused by the combination of wind, fire, phlegm and deficiency. It is worth noting that in the book *Lei Zheng Pu Ji Ben Shi Fang Shi Yi* 类证普济本事方释义 (1750 AD), clinicians recorded that the disease *tou feng* 头风 was more prevalent in female patients and it was caused by Blood deficiency combined with wind invasion in the Liver meridian.

Similar explanations of the aetiology of migraine were also recorded in two books published in the Qing dynasty (1645–1911 AD), *Za Bing Yuan Liu Xi Zhu* 杂病源流犀烛•头痛源流 (1773 AD) and *Zhang Shi Yi Tong* 张氏医通•诸痛门 (1695 AD). In addition, *qi* stagnation in combination with wind invasion in the *Shao yang* 少阳 meridian can also cause migraine, as recorded in the book *Bian Zheng Lun* 辨证录 (1687 AD). In summary, it was traditionally believed that migraine was a disease due to problems that occurred in *Shao yang* 少阳, *Yang ming* 阳明 and foot *Jue yin* 厥阴 meridians; it could be caused by both external pathogens (wind, cold, fire and heat) and internal pathogens (phlegm and *qi*), with wind invasion being the leading factor.

Chinese Medicine Syndromes

As stated above, migraine was believed to be caused by a combination of external pathogens (wind, cold, fire and heat) and internal pathogens (phlegm and *qi*) and the meridian-determined pain location also play an important role in migraine's syndrome differentiation. Chinese medicine clinical treatments for migraine should take all these factors into consideration. Chinese herbal medicine treatment may work on resolving the pathogenesis based on syndrome differentiation, with the assistance of some herbs leading the therapeutic effects to certain meridians; acupuncture-related therapies may be targeting particular symptoms in combination with treatment based on syndrome differentiation.

Chinese Herbal Medicine

The 1,514 citations describing CHM treatments were identified in 240 books. Books with the largest yield of citations included *Pu Ji Fang* 普济方 (1406 AD) (*n* = 199), *Sheng Ji Zong Lu* 圣济总录 (1117 AD) (*n* = 52), *Ji Yang Gang Mu* 济阳纲目 (1626 AD) (*n* = 52), *Ben Cao Gang Mu* 本草纲目 (1578 AD) (*n* = 45) and *Zheng Zhi Zhun Sheng* 证治准绳 (1602 AD) (*n* = 45). Thirty-nine books obtained ten or more included citations of CHM treatment.

Frequency of Treatment Citations by Dynasty

The majority of citations with CHM treatments were found from the classical books published in the Ming dynasty (1369–1644 AD) and the Qing dynasty (1645–1911 AD) (Table 3.4). Around 80% of citations (*n* = 1,207)

Table 3.4.   Dynastic Distribution of Treatment Citations

Dynasty	No. of Treatment Citations
Before Tang dynasty (before 618 AD)	11
Tang and 5 dynasties (618–960 AD)	4
Song and Jin dynasties (961–1271 AD)	199
Yuan dynasty (1272–1368 AD)	62
Ming dynasty (1369–1644 AD)	636
Qing dynasty (1645–1911 AD)	571
Ming Guo/Republic of China (1912–1949 AD)	30
Japan	1
Total	1,514

were identified during this period. One citation was found in classical literature published in Japan during the Qing dynasty.

The earliest citations with CHM treatments (*n* = 2) were identified in *Jin Kui Yao Lue* 金匮要略 (219 AD). These two citations were found by the search terms *tou feng* 头风 and *tou tong* 头痛. One citation suggested an oral CHM formula, *Wu zhu yu tang* 吴茱萸汤, and another one introduced topical CHM, *Tou feng mo san* 头风摩散.

The latest citations (*n* = 10) stated that CHM formulas were found in *Ben Cao Jian Yao Fang* 本草简要方 (1938 AD) published in the Ming Guo period (1912–1949 AD). A number of formulas were described to treat migraine either orally or topically, including *Xi xin tang* 细辛汤, *Jing jie san* 荆芥散 and *Yi ping wan* 一品丸. One citation described the CM pathogenesis of *pian tou feng* 偏头风 as '*pian tou feng* 偏头风, if symptoms occur on the left side are caused by Blood deficiency, while symptoms on the right side are caused by excessive heat of *qi* 偏头风, 左为血虚, 右为气热'.

Treatment with Chinese Herbal Medicine

The 1,514 CHM treatment citations were all considered 'possibly' related to migraine as they met the inclusion criteria. Of these, a total of 178 citations were judged as the 'most likely' migraine citations following the criteria as mentioned above. Data extracted from the originated 'possible' migraine citations dataset and 'most likely' migraine citations sub-dataset were analysed for frequently used formulas and herbs.

Most Frequent Formulas in 'Possible' Migraine Citations

A total of 1,534 formulas were identified from the 'possible' migraine citations dataset, with 692 (45.2%) citations that did not provide formula names. The majority of the formulas were described for oral use (*n* = 1,022; 66.6%) and 512 (33.4%) CHM formulas were for topical use.

The most frequently cited oral formula names and their herb ingredients are presented in Table 3.5. Herbal ingredients were

Table 3.5. Most Frequent Oral Formulas in 'Possible' Migraine Citations

Formula Name	Herb Ingredients	Number of Citations (*n*)
Qing kong gao 清空膏	*Chuan xiong* 川芎, *chai hu* 柴胡, *huang lian* 黄连, *fang feng* 防风, *qiang huo* 羌活, *zhi gan cao* 炙甘草, *huang qin* 黄芩 and *cha* 茶. (*Ren Zhai Zhi Zhi Fang Lun* 仁斋直指方论, 1264 AD)	32
Chuan xiong cha tiao san 川芎茶调散	*Bo he* 薄荷, *chuan xiong* 川芎, *jing jie* 荆芥, *xiang fu* 香附, *fang feng* 防风, *bai zhi* 白芷, *jiang huo* 羌活, *gan cao* 甘草 and *cha* 茶. (*Tai Ping Hui Min He Ji Ju Fang* 太平惠民和剂局方, 1107 AD)	27
Chuan xiong san 川芎散	*Chuan xiong* 川芎, *xi xin* 细辛, *qiang huo* 羌活, *huai hua* 槐花, *shi gao* 石膏, *xiang fu* 香附, *gan cao* 甘草, *jing jie* 荆芥, *bo he* 薄荷, *yin chen* 茵陈, *fang feng* 防风, *ju hua* 菊花 and *cha* 茶. (*Wei Sheng Bao Jian* 卫生宝鉴, 1343 AD)	20
Cha tiao san 茶调散	*Ju hua* 菊花, *xi xin* 细辛, *shi gao* 石膏, *xiang fu* 香附 and *cha* 茶. (*Sheng Ji Zong Lu* 圣济总录, 1117 AD)	17
Xiong xi wan 芎犀丸	*Shi gao* 石膏, *bing pian* 冰片, *zhu sha* 朱砂, *niu xi* 牛犀, *ren shen* 人参, *fu ling* 茯苓, *chuan xiong* 川芎, *e jiao* 阿胶, *xi xin* 细辛, *mai men dong* 麦门冬, *gan cao* 甘草, *zhi zi* 栀子, *mi* 蜜, *cha* 茶 and *jiu* 酒. (*Shi Yi De Xiao Fang* 世医得效方, 1345 AD)	14
Zhui feng san 追风散	*Long gu* 龙骨, *wu gong* 蜈蚣, *chi xiao dou* 赤小豆, *hu gu* 虎骨, *jiang chan* 僵蚕, *cao wu* 草乌, *bai jiao xiang* 白胶香, *tian ma* 天麻, *chuan xiu xi* 川牛膝, *dang gui* 当归, *quan xie* 全蝎, *ru xiang* 乳香, *mu bie* 木鳖, *cu* 醋, *cha* 茶 and *jiu* 酒. (*Tai Ping Hui Min He Ji Ju Fang* 太平惠民和剂局方, 1107 AD)	14
Da chuan xiong wan 大川芎丸	*Chuan xiong* 川芎 and *tian ma* 天麻. (*Sheng Ji Zong Lu* 圣济总录, 1117 AD)	11
Du liang wan 都梁丸	*Bai zhi* 白芷, *mi* 蜜 and *cha* 茶. (*Yan Shi Ji Sheng Fang* 严氏济生方, 1253 AD)	11

Table 3.5.   (*Continued*)

Formula Name	Herb Ingredients	Number of Citations (*n*)
Wu zhu yu tang 吴茱萸汤	*Ren shen* 人参, *wu zhu yu* 吴茱萸, *sheng jiang* 生姜 and *zhao* 枣. (*Jin Gui Yao Lue Fang Lun* 金匮要略方论, 219 AD)	10
Ru xiang zhan luo san 乳香盏落散	*Ying su ke* 罂粟壳, *chai hu* 柴胡, *jie geng* 桔梗, *gan cao* 甘草 and *chen pi* 陈皮. (*Wei Sheng Bao Jian* 卫生宝鉴, 1343 AD)	9
Ru sheng bing zi 如圣饼子	*Chuan wu* 川乌, *tian nan xing* 天南星, *gan jiang* 干姜, *gan cao* 甘草, *chuan xiong* 川芎, *fang feng* 防风, *tian ma* 天麻, *jing jie* 荆芥 and *cha* 茶. (*Ji Feng Pu Ji Fang* 鸡峰普济方, 1133 AD)	9
Yu zhen wan 玉真丸	*Liu huang* 硫黄, *shi gao* 石膏, *ban xia* 半夏, *mang xiao* 芒硝 and *sheng jiang* 生姜. (*Ye Shi Lu Yan Fang* 叶氏录验方, 1186 AD)	9
Shi gao san 石膏散	*Shi gao* 石膏, *chuan xiong* 川芎, *gan cao* 甘草, *cong* 葱 and *cha* 茶. (*Sheng Ji Zong Lu* 圣济总录, 1117 AD)	9
Xiong xin tang 芎辛汤	*Fu zi* 附子, *wu tou* 乌头, *tian nan xing* 天南星, *gan jiang* 干姜, *gan cao* 甘草, *chuan xiong* 川芎, xi xin 细辛, *sheng jiang* 生姜 and cha 茶. (*San Yin Ji Yi Bing Zheng Fang Lun* 三因极一病证方论, 1174 AD)	9

1. Formula ingredients are based on the earliest book within the group of included citations.

2. Formulas with the same name can vary in their ingredients, and the same combination of ingredients may have different names. In this data, formulas with the same name that have variations in a few ingredients are grouped together, while those large variations in ingredients are separated. Also, formulas with the same ingredients but different names have been grouped together.

3. The use of some herbs/ingredients may be restricted in some countries, e.g. herbs such as *xi xin* 细辛 and *ying su ke* 罂粟壳 can be toxic or addictive. Readers are advised to comply with relevant regulations.

obtained from the earliest citation if variants were seen under the same formula name. Consistent with the current management for migraine, three most frequent cited oral formulas *Chuan xiong cha tiao san* 川芎茶调散, *Wu zhu yu tang* 吴茱萸汤, and *Da chuan xiong wan* 大川芎丸 are also recommended in contemporary CM guide-lines[10] and textbooks.[9]

Qing kong gao 清空膏 was the most frequently described formula to treat migraine orally. The earliest citation cited, *Qing kong gao* 清空膏 was obtained from *Ren Zhai Zhi Zhi Fang Lun* 仁斋直指方论 (1264 AD). Herbal ingredients were formulated to carry the functions of clearing heat, expelling wind and relieving pain, which is consistent with the treatment principle against hyperactivity of Liver *yang* in contemporary CM guidelines[10] and textbooks[9].

Three oral formulas sharing similar formula names, *Chuan xiong cha tiao san* 川芎茶调散, *Chuan xiong san* 川芎散 and *Cha tiao san* 茶调散, were identified in this dataset. It should be noted that *Chuan xiong cha tiao san* 川芎茶调散 and *Chuan xiong san* 川芎散 were also similar in terms of herbal ingredients; these two formulas may refer to one formula with different Chinese names, with *Chuan xiong san* 川芎散 serving as a shorted name of *Chuan xiong cha tiao san* 川芎茶调散. However, differences were seen in the ingredients of *Cha tiao san* 茶调散 when compared with the other two formulas, suggesting that *Cha tiao san* 茶调散 was used as a different formula in ancient times.

One oral formula, *Ru xiang zhan luo san* 乳香盏落散, contains the name of the herb *ru xiang* 乳香 in the formula name. However, *ru xiang* 乳香 has not been identified as one ingredient used in the formula. Typographical error may be one possible reason when the ancient authors were creating the transcription of the literature.

The most frequently cited topical formula found in the 'possible' migraine citations was *Tou ding san* 透顶散, identified from 13 cita-tions (Table 3.6). The earliest citation of this formula was obtained in *Lei Zheng Pu Ji Ben Shi Fang Xu Ji* 类证普济本事方续集 (1132 AD). These CHM formulas were applied as sniffing or external application. Although many topical formulas were cited in classical literature, the contemporary CM textbooks recommend only several unnamed for-mulas for migraine. It may suggest that topical CHM treatment was more popular to manage migraine in ancient times than currently.

Table 3.6.   Most Frequent Topical Formulas in 'Possible' Migraine Citations

Formula Name	Herb Ingredients	Number of Citations (*n*)
Tou ding san 透顶散	*Xi xin* 细辛, *gua di* 瓜蒂, *ding xiang* 丁香, *nao zi* 脑子 and *she xiang* 麝香. (*Lei zheng pu ji ben shi fang xu ji* 类证普济本事方续集, 1132 AD)	13
Tou feng mo san 头风摩散	*Fu zi* 附子 and *yan* 盐. (*Jin Kui Yao Lue Fang Lun* 金匮要略方论, 219AD)	10
Zhi ling san 至灵散	*Xiong huang* 雄黄 and *xi xin* 细辛. (*Zhou hou bei ji fang* 肘后备急方, 363 AD)	9
Tou ding san 通顶散	*Bing pian* 冰片, *di long* 地龙, *gua di* 瓜蒂, *chi xiao dou* 赤小豆 and *mang xiao* 芒硝. (*Sheng ji zong lu* 圣济总录, 1117 AD)	8
Long xiang san 龙香散	*Di long* 地龙 and *ru xiang* 乳香. (*Pu ji fang* 普济方, 1406 AD)	6
Bi ba san 荜茇散	*Bi ba* 荜茇. (*Sheng ji zong lu* 圣济总录, 1117 AD)	5
Yi di jin 一滴金	*Ren zhong bai* 人中白, *di long* 地龙 and *yang dan zhi* 羊胆汁. (*Sheng ji zong lu* 圣济总录, 1117 AD)	4
Ding xiang san 丁香散	*Ding xiang* 丁香, *ji zhen* 棘针 and *she xiang* 麝香. (*Sheng ji zong lu* 圣济总录, 1117 AD)	3
Gua di shen miao san 瓜蒂神妙散	*Yan xiao* 焰硝, *xiong huang* 雄黄, *chuan xiong* 川芎, *bo he* 薄荷, *cang er zi* 苍耳子, *li lu* 藜芦 and *tian zhu huang* 天竺黄. (*Huang di su wen xuan ming lun fang* 黄帝素问宣明论方, 1172 AD)	3
Zi jin ding 紫金锭	*Shan ci gu* 山慈菇, *wen ge* 文蛤, *she xiang* 麝香, *qian jin zi* 千金子, *da ji* 大戟, *nuo mi* 糯米 and *bo he* 薄荷. (*Yi xue ru men* 医学入门, 1575 AD)	3
Tong tian san 通天散	*Chi shao* 赤芍, *chuan xiong* 川芎, *huang lian* 黄连, *huang qin* 黄芩, *yan hu suo* 延胡索, *cao wu* 草乌, *dang gui* 当归 and *ru xiang* 乳香. (*Huang di su wen xuan ming lun fang* 黄帝素问宣明论方, 172 AD)	3

1. Formula ingredients are based on the earliest book within the group of included citations.

2. Formulas with the same name can vary in their ingredients, and the same combination of ingredients may have different names. In this data, formulas with the same name that have variations in a few ingredients are grouped together, while those with large variations in ingredients are separated. Also, formulas with the same ingredients but different names have been grouped together.

3. The use of some herbs/ingredients may be restricted in some countries, e.g. herbs such as *xi xin* 细辛 can be toxic and some herbs e.g. *she xiang* 麝香 may be restricted under the Convention on International Trade in Endangered Species of Wild Fauna and Flora (CITES). Readers are advised to comply with relevant regulations.

Most Frequent Herbs in 'Possible' Migraine Citations

Of these included citations, a total of 350 ingredients were identified for oral use. Some ingredients with different Chinese names or preparation methods but similar clinical functions were merged for frequency analysis. The most frequently reported orally used ingredient was *chuan xiong* 川芎, obtained from 519 citations (Table 3.7). *Chuan xiong* 川芎 is the key herb used in multiple frequently used

Table 3.7.   Most Frequent Oral Herbs in 'Possible' Migraine Citations

Herb Name	Scientific Name	No. of Citations (*n*)
Chuan xiong 川芎	*Ligusticum chuanxiong* Hort.	519
Gan cao/zhi gan cao/ sheng gan cao 甘草/炙甘草/生甘草	*Glycyrrhizae spp.*	411 (362/32/17)
Cha 茶	Tea	401
Chuan wu/cao wu/wu tou/fu zi/sheng fu zi/shu fu zi 川乌/草乌/乌头/附子/生附子/熟附子	*Aconitum carmichaeli* Debx.	322 (146/70/37/66/2/1)
Fang feng 防风	*Saposhnikovia divaricata* (Turcz.) Schischk.	275
Sheng jiang/gan jiang/ jiang/pao jiang 生姜/干姜/姜/炮姜	*Zingiber officinale* (Willd.) Rosc.	262 (198/61/1/2)
Bai zhi 白芷	*Angelica dahurica* (Fisch. ex Hoffm.) Benth.& Hook. f.	253
Jing jie/jing jie sui 荆芥/荆芥穗	*Schizonepeta tenuifolia* (Benth.) Briq.	233 (161/72)
Xi xin 细辛	1. *Asarum heterotropoides* Fr. Schmidt var. mandshuricum (Maxim) Kitag. 2. *Asarum sieboldii* Miq. var. seoulense Nakai 3. *Asarum sieboldii* Miq.	222
Bo he 薄荷	*Mentha haplocalyx* Briq.	211

Table 3.7. (*Continued*)

Herb Name	Scientific Name	No. of Citations (*n*)
Qiang huo 羌活	*Notopterygium incisum* Ting	195
Jiu 酒	Wine	195
Shi gao 石膏	Crystalline gypsum (calcium sulphate)	175
Tian ma 天麻	*Gastrodia elata* Bl.	165
Ban xia/ban xia qu/fa ban xia/zhi ban xia/sheng ban xia 半夏/半夏曲/法半夏/制半夏/生半夏	*Pinellia ternata* (Thunb.) Breit.	160 (141/10/5/3/1)
Tian nan xing/dan nan xing 天南星/胆南星	*Arisaema consanguineum* Schott	150 (143/7)
Dang gui/dang gui shen/ dang gui wei 当归/当归身/当归尾	*Angelica sinensis* (Oliv.) Diels.	148 (142/5/1)
Huang qin 黄芩	*Scutellaria baicalensis* Georgi.	120
Ju hua 菊花	*Chrysanthemum morifolium* Ramat.	118
Fu ling/fu shen 茯苓/茯神	*Poria cocos* (Schw.) Wolf.	116 (104/12)

The use of some herbs/ingredients may be restricted in some countries, e.g. herbs such as *wu tou* 乌头 and *fu zi* 附子 can be toxic. Readers are advised to comply with relevant regulations.

oral formulas such as *Qing kong gao* 清空膏, *Chuan xiong cha tiao san* 川芎茶调散, *Chuan xiong san* 川芎散 and *Da chuan xiong wan* 大川芎丸. *Chuan xiong* 川芎 is used to activate Blood, regulate *qi*, expel wind and relieve pain in CHM practice, which is beneficial for relieving migraine symptoms. Most of the other frequently reported herbs have the functions of expelling cold and wind and relieving pain, which is consistent with the aetiology of migraine.

A total of 229 ingredients were reported for topical use in the included citations. The most frequently reported topical ingredients included *xi xin* 细辛 (85 citations), *mang xiao* 芒硝 (61 citations) and *she xiang* 麝香 (57 citations). These ingredients all carry the function of relieving pain (Table 3.8). It is noted that many of these topically

Table 3.8.   Most Frequent Topical Herbs in 'Possible' Migraine Citations

Herb Name	Scientific Name	No. of Citations (*n*)
Xi xin 细辛	1. *Asarum heterotropoides* Fr. Schmidt var. mandshuricum (Maxim) Kitag. 2. *Asarum sieboldii* Miq. var. seoulense Nakai 3. *Asarum sieboldii* Miq.	85
Mang xiao/xiao shi/yan xiao/xi gua xiao 芒硝/硝石/焰硝/西瓜硝	Mirabilite	61 (30/24/5/2)
She xiang 麝香	*Moschus moschiferus* Linnaeus	57
Ru xiang 乳香	*Boswellia carterii* Birdw.	54
Chuan xiong 川芎	*Ligusticum chuanxiong* Hort.	52
Lai fu/lai fu zhi/lai fu zi/lai fu pi 莱菔/莱菔汁/莱菔子/莱菔皮	*Raphanus sativus* L.	51 (2/43/5/1)
Bing pian/nao zi 冰片/脑子	1. *Dryobalanops aromatica* Gaertn. 2. *Blumea balsamifera* DC.	47 (24/23)
Cao wu/chuan wu/wu tou/fu zi 草乌/川乌/乌头/附子	*Aconitum carmichaeli* Debx.	48(18/15/1/14)
Bai zhi 白芷	*Angelica dahurica* (Fisch.ex Hoffm.) Benth.& Hook. f.	44
Bi ma zi 蓖麻子	*Ricinus communis* L.	44
Xiong huang 雄黄	Realgar	39
Gua di 瓜蒂	*Cucumis melo* L.	34
Yan 盐	Salt	33
Bi ba 荜茇	*Piper longum* L.	32
Di long 地龙	*Pheretima aspergillum* (Perrier)	26
Sheng jiang/sheng jiang zhi/gan jiang 生姜/生姜汁/干姜	*Zingiber officinale* (Willd.) Rosc.	25 (12/9/4)
Zao jia 皂荚	*Gleditsia sinensis* Lam.	24
Bo he 薄荷	*Mentha haplocalyx* Briq.	24

The use of some herbs/ingredients may be restricted in some countries, e.g. herbs such as *xi xin* 细辛, *wu tou* 乌头 and *fu zi* 附子 can be toxic, and some herbs e.g. *she xiang* 麝香 may be restricted under the Convention on International Trade in Endangered Species of Wild Fauna and Flora (CITES). Readers are advised to comply with relevant regulations.

used herbs were also frequently used orally. For example, *chuan xiong* 川芎 is the most frequently used oral herb, as well as one of the most cited herbs for topical use (52 citations), suggesting its importance in managing this disease.

Most Frequent Formulas in 'Most Likely' Migraine Citations

A total of 178 citations containing CHM treatments were further judged as 'mostly likely' to be migraine. Among these, around two thirds of CHM formulas were for oral use ($n = 112$; 62.9%), 64 formulas were reported to be used topically, and two formulas were used both orally and topically. There were 59 CHM treatments considered as CHM formulas because they used a group of herbs, although there was not a formula name provided by the book.

The oral and topical formulas identified in two or more citations are listed in Tables 3.9 and 3.10, respectively. Six of the most frequent

Table 3.9. Most Frequent Oral Formulas in 'Most Likely' Migraine Citations

Formula Name	Herb Ingredients	No. of Citations (*n*)
Qing kong gao 清空膏	*Chuan xiong* 川芎, *chai hu* 柴胡, *huang lian* 黄连, *fang feng* 防风, *qiang huo* 羌活, *zhi gan cao* 炙甘草, *huang qin* 黃芩 and *cha* 茶. (*Ren zhai zhi zhi fang lun* 仁斋直指方论, 1264 AD)	17
Zhui feng san 追风散	*Long gu* 龙骨, *wu gong* 蜈蚣, *chi xiao dou* 赤小豆, *hu gu* 虎骨, *jiang chan* 僵蚕, *cao wu* 草乌, *bai jiao xiang* 白胶香, *tian ma* 天麻, *chuan xiu xi* 川牛膝, *dang gui* 当归, *quan xie* 全蝎, *ru xiang* 乳香, *mu bie* 木鳖, *cu* 醋, *cha* 茶 and *jiu* 酒. (*Tai ping hui min he ji ju fang* 太平惠民和剂局方, 1107 AD)	7
Ru xiang zhan luo san 乳香盏落散	*Ying su ke* 罂粟壳, *chai hu* 柴胡, *jie geng* 桔梗, *gan cao* 甘草 and *chen pi* 陈皮. (*Wei sheng bao jian* 卫生宝鉴, 1343 AD)	6
Ru sheng bing zi 如圣饼子	*Chuan wu* 川乌, *tian nan xing* 天南星, *gan jiang* 干姜, *gan cao* 甘草, *chuan xiong* 川芎, *fang feng* 防风, *tian ma* 天麻, *jing jie* 荆芥 and *cha* 茶. (*Ji feng pu ji fang* 鸡峰普济方, 1133 AD)	6

(Continued)

Table 3.9. (*Continued*)

Formula Name	Herb Ingredients	No. of Citations (*n*)
Ren shen ban xia wan 人参半夏丸	*Ren shen* 人参, *fu ling* 茯苓, *bo he* 薄荷, *tian nan xing* 天南星, *han shui shi* 寒水石, *bai fan* 白矾, *gan jiang* 干姜, *ban xia* 半夏, *ge fen* 蛤粉, *huo xiang* 藿香, *mian* 面 and *sheng jiang* 生姜. (*Yu yao yuan fang* 御药院方, 1267 AD)	5
Xiong xin tang 芎辛汤	*Fu zi* 附子, *wu tou* 乌头, *tian nan xing* 天南星, *gan jiang* 干姜, *gan cao* 甘草, *chuan xiong* 川芎, *xi xin* 细辛, *sheng jiang* 生姜, and *cha* 茶. (*San yin ji yi bing zheng fang lun* 三因极一病证方论, 1174 AD)	4
Da fu wan 大附丸	*Fu zi* 附子, *cong* 葱 and *cha* 茶. (*San yin ji yi bing zheng fang lun* 三因极一病证方论, 1174 AD)	2
Tai yi zi jin dan 太乙紫金丹	*Da ji* 大戟, *shan ci gu* 山慈菇, *wen ge* 文蛤, *she xiang* 麝香, *zhu sha* 朱砂, *qian jin zi* 千金子, *xiong huang* 雄黄 and *nuo mi* 糯米. (*Wai ke zheng zong* 外科正宗, 1617 AD)	2
Bi sheng san 必胜散	*Fu zi* 附子, *gao liang jiang* 高良姜 and *cha* 茶. (*Pu ji fang* 普济方, 1406 AD)	2
Shi gao wan 石膏丸	*Shi gao* 石膏, *xuan jing shi* 玄精石, *mang xiao* 芒硝, *wu tou* 乌头, *sheng jiang* 生姜 and *jing jie* 荆芥. (*Ji feng pu ji fang* 鸡峰普济方, 1133 AD)	2
Kong qing gao 空青膏	*Qiang huo* 羌活, *fang feng* 防风, *huang lian* 黄连, *gan cao* 甘草, *chai hu* 柴胡, *chuan xiong* 川芎, *huang qin* 黄芩 and *cha* 茶. (*Jian ming yi gou* 简明医彀, 1629 AD)	2
Cha tiao san 茶调散	*Ju hua* 菊花, *xi xin* 细辛, *shi gao* 石膏, *xiang fu* 香附 and *cha* 茶. (*Sheng ji zong lu* 圣济总录, 1117 AD)	2
Huang niu nao sui jiu 黄牛脑髓酒	*Niu nao* 牛脑, *bai zhi* 白芷, *chuan xiong* 川芎 and *jiu* 酒. (*Yi xue ru men* 医学入门, 1575 AD)	2

1. Formula ingredients are based on the earliest book within the group of included citations.

2. Formulas with the same name can vary in their ingredients, and the same combination of ingredients may have different names. In this data, formulas with the same name that have variations in a few ingredients are grouped together while those large variations in ingredients are separated. Also, formulas with the same ingredients but different names have been grouped together.

3. The use of some herbs/ingredients may be restricted in some countries. For example, herbs such as *xi xin* 细辛, *wu tou* 乌头 and *fu zi* 附子 can be toxic, and *ying su ke* 罂粟壳 is addictive. Some other herbs e.g. *she xiang* 麝香 may be restricted under the Convention on International Trade in Endangered Species of Wild Fauna and Flora (CITES). Readers are advised to comply with relevant regulations.

Table 3.10.   Most Frequent Topical Formulas in 'Most Likely' Migraine Citations

Formula Name	Herb Ingredients	No. of Citations (*n*)
Tou ding san 透顶散	*Xi xin* 细辛, *gua di* 瓜蒂, *ding xiang* 丁香, *nao zi* 脑子 and *she xiang* 麝香. (*Lei zheng pu ji ben shi fang xu ji* 类证普济本事方续集, 1132 AD)	11
Tong ding san 通顶散	*Bing pian* 冰片, *di long* 地龙, *gua di* 瓜蒂, *chi xiao dou* 赤小豆 and *mang xiao* 芒硝. (*Sheng ji zong lu* 圣济总录, 1117 AD)	3
Long xiang san 龙香散	*Di long* 地龙 and *ru xiang* 乳香. (*Pu ji fang* 普济方, 1406 AD)	3

1. Formula ingredients are based on the earliest book within the group of included citations.

2. Formulas with the same name can vary in their ingredients, and the same combination of ingredients may have different names. In this data, formulas with the same name that have variations in a few ingredients are grouped together while those large variations in ingredients are separated. Also, formulas with the same ingredients but different names have been grouped together.

3. The use of some herbs/ingredients may be restricted in some countries, e.g. herbs such as *xi xin* 细辛 can be toxic and some other herbs e.g. *she xiang* 麝香 may be restricted under the Convention on International Trade in Endangered Species of Wild Fauna and Flora (CITES). Readers are advised to comply with relevant regulations.

oral formulas in 'most likely' migraine citations also appeared in the 'possible' migraine citations most frequently cited formula list, including *Qing kong gao* 清空膏, *Cha tiao san* 茶调散, *Zhui feng san* 追风散, *Ru xiang zhan luo san* 乳香盏落散, *Ru sheng bing zi* 如圣饼子 and *Xiong xin tang* 芎辛汤. The clinical functions of these most frequently used formulas are similar, including expelling wind, regulating *qi* and resolving pain, which is consistent with the contemporary treatment principle for migraine in CM theory.

Three topical formulas were found in more than two citations. These formulae were also found in the 'possible' migraine citations most frequently reported formula pool, confirming the use of topical CHM for this clinical condition in history.

Most Frequent Herbs in 'Most Likely' Migraine Citations

The formulas obtained from the 'most likely' migraine citations were further analysed for the ingredients. A total of 128 herbs were identified as oral use, while 64 herbs were identified for topical use. The top 20 most frequently reported oral and topical herbs are presented in Tables 3.11 and 3.12, respectively. Similar to formulas, these most frequently used oral and topical herbs in 'most likely'

Table 3.11.   Most Frequent Oral Herbs in 'Most Likely' Migraine Citations

Herb Name	Scientific Name	No. of Citations (*n*)
Gan cao/zhi gan cao/Sheng gan cao 甘草/炙甘草/生甘草	*Glycyrrhizae spp.*	63 (50/10/3)
Chuan xiong 川芎	*Ligusticum chuanxiong* Hort.	60
Cha 茶	Tea	58
Chuan wu/cao wu/wu tou/fu zi/sheng fu zi/hei fu zi 川乌/草乌/乌头/附子/生附子/黑附子	*Aconitum carmichaeli* Debx.	56 (20/17/5/11/2/1)
Fang feng 防风	*Saposhnikovia divaricata* (Turcz.) Schischk.	47
Sheng jiang/gan jiang 生姜/干姜	*Zingiber officinale* (Willd.) Rosc.	41 (23/18)
Qiang huo 羌活	*Notopterygium incisum* Ting	32
Tian nan xing 天南星	*Arisaema consanguineum* Schott	31
Chai hu 柴胡	*Bupleurum chinense* DC.	30
Tian ma 天麻	*Gastrodia elata* Bl.	25
Huang qin 黄芩	*Scutellaria baicalensis* Georgi	24
Huang lian 黄连	*Coptis chinensis* Franch.	24
Ban xia/fa ban xia/sheng ban xia 半夏/法半夏/生半夏	*Pinellia ternata* (Thunb.) Breit.	24 (22/1/1)
Bai zhi 白芷	*Angelica dahurica* (Fisch.ex Hoffm.) Benth.& Hook. f.	22
Jiu 酒	Wine	21
Jing jie/jing jie sui 荆芥/荆芥穗	*Schizonepeta tenuifolia* (Benth.) Briq.	21 (12/9)

Table 3.11. (*Continued*)

Herb Name	Scientific Name	No. of Citations (*n*)
Xi xin 细辛	1. *Asarum heterotropoides* Fr. Schmidt var. mandshuricum (Maxim) Kitag. 2. *Asarum sieboldii* Miq. var. seoulense Nakai 3. *Asarum sieboldii* Miq.	18
Chen pi/qing pi/ju hong 陈皮/青皮/橘红	*Citrus reticulata* Blanco	18 (15/1/2)
Shi gao 石膏	Crystalline gypsum (calcium sulphate)	16
Jiang can 僵蚕	1. *Bombyx mori* L. 2. *Beauveria bassiana* (Bals) Vuill.	14
Quan xie/xie shao 全蝎/蝎梢	*Buthus martensi* Karsch	14 (13/1)

The use of some herbs/ingredients may be restricted in some countries. For example, herbs such as *xi xin* 细辛, *wu tou* 乌头 and *fu zi* 附子 can be toxic. Readers are advised to comply with relevant regulations.

Table 3.12. Most Frequent Topical Herbs in 'Most Likely' Migraine Citations

Herb Name	Scientific Name	No. of Citations (*n*)
Gua di 瓜蒂	*Cucumis melo* L.	16
Xi xin 细辛	1. *Asarum heterotropoides* Fr. Schmidt var. mandshuricum (Maxim) Kitag. 2. *Asarum sieboldii* Miq. var. seoulense Nakai 3. *Asarum sieboldii* Miq.	15
She xiang 麝香	*Moschus moschiferus* Linnaeus	15
Nao zi/bing pian 脑子/冰片	1. *Dryobalanops aromatica* Gaertn. 2. *Blumea balsamifera* DC.	15 (9/6)
Ding xiang 丁香	*Syzygium aromaticum* (L.) Merr. et Perry	11
Ru xiang 乳香	*Boswellia carterii* Birdw.	9
Nuo mi 糯米	*Oryza sativa* L. var. glutinosa	9

(*Continued*)

Table 3.12.   (*Continued*)

Herb Name	Scientific Name	No. of Citations (*n*)
Lai fu zhi/lai fu/lai fu zi 莱菔汁/莱菔/莱菔子	*Raphanus sativus* L.	8 (6/1/1)
Di long 地龙	*Pheretima aspergillum* (Perrier)	7
Mang xiao 芒硝	Mirabilite	6
Bi ma zi 蓖麻子	*Ricinus communis* L.	6
Jiu 酒	Wine	6
Yan hu suo 延胡索	*Corydalis yanhusuo* W.T. Wang	5
Zhao jia 皂荚	*Gleditsia sinensis* Lam.	5
Zao 枣	*Ziziphus jujuba* Mill. var. inermis (Bge.) Rehd.	4
Bi ba 荜茇	*Piper longum* L.	4
Xiong huang 雄黄	Realgar	4
Qing dai 青黛	1. *Baphicacanthus cusia* (Nees) Brem 2. *Indigofera tinctoria* L. 3. *Isatis tinctoria* L. 4. *Isatis indigotica* Fort. 5. *Polygonum tinctorium* Ait.	4
Gui xin/rou gui 桂心/肉桂	*Cinnamomum cassia* Presl	4 (3/1)

The use of some herbs/ingredients may be restricted in some countries. For example, herbs such as *xi xin* 细辛 can be toxic. Some other herbs e.g. *she xiang* 麝香 may be restricted under the Convention on International Trade in Endangered Species of Wild Fauna and Flora (CITES). Readers are advised to comply with relevant regulations.

migraine citations were consistent with the herb pools obtained from 'possible' migraine citations. The functions of these most frequent herbs/ingredients include tonifying *qi* and *yang*, relieving pain, expelling wind and phlegm, regulating *qi*, clearing heat and activating Blood, which are consistent with the complex aetiology of migraine according to contemporary guidelines. As different herbs were to be formulated based on syndrome differentiations, a wide range of herbs/ingredients with different functions were identified in these pools.

Chinese Herbal Medicine Used Both Orally and Topically (in the 'Most Likely' Pool)

Two citations of 'most likely' migraine used the same herbs both orally and topically. One citation was identified from *Pu Ji Fang* 普济方 (1390 AD), stating that ground *cong* 葱 (spring onion) mixed with alcohol, can be taken orally and also applied on the temple region to treat chronic *pian zheng tou feng* 偏正头风 (年深月远, 头脑疼胀, 太阳跳痛, 偏正头风及杨梅愈后余毒入注, 脑门作痛, 俱用葱, 酒磨服, 兼涂太阳). The other citation was found from *Tong Yuan Yi Shu* 彤园医书 (1795 AD) introducing the powder of *bi bo* 荜茇 which can be taken orally with tea and also sniffed into the nose to treat severe chronic migraine (荜茇散 (出杨氏家藏方). 治年深头风, 痰厥呕吐, 恶闻人声, 头不能举, 目不能开, 荜茇（不以多少）上为细末, 每服一大钱, 茶清调下, 仍搐少许鼻中, 食后).

Representative Citations

One citation, identified from a book published in the Jin 晋 dynasty (266–420 AD), *Zhou Hou Bei Ji Fang* 肘后备急方 (363 AD), stated that 'the CHM formula *Zhi Ling San* 至灵散 can be used to treat *pian tou teng* 偏头疼: Grind CHM herbs *xiong huang* 雄黄 and *xi xin* 细辛 to be fine powder, sniff it into nostril when headache occurs'. Such therapy is still in use in current clinical practice. However, in this book, the advice was to 'sniff CHM into the right nostril to treat left-side headache, sniff CHM into the left nostril to treat right-side headache'; this left-right practice is not included in contemporary literature. Another citation identified from *Jing Yan Hou Fang* 经验后方, a book published at a similar time, also suggested CHM sniffing powder to treat *pian tou teng* 偏头疼: sniff *bi ba* 荜茇 powder into the right nostril to treat left-side headache, and vice versa.

In the books published in the Song dynasty (961–1271 AD), the disease *pian tou teng* 偏头疼 was described with more details in terms of accompanying symptoms. For example, in the book *San Yin Ji Yi Bing Zheng Fang Lun* 三因极一病证方论 (1174 AD), oral CHM formula *Ru sheng bing zi* 如圣饼子 was used to treat *pian zheng tou teng* 偏正头疼, which is 'a condition caused by pathogens stagnated in *yang* meridians presenting with headache reaching the top of head, vomiting and nausea, accompanied by loss of vision and hearing …'. In the book *Yan Shi Ji Sheng Fang* 严氏济生方 (1253 AD), *pian zheng tou teng* 偏正头疼 was treated by *Er qiong bing zi* 二芎饼子, with similar symptoms described. An oral CHM formula, *Qing kong gao* 清空膏, was suggested to treat long-term severe *pian zheng tou tong* 偏正头痛 which impacts vision in the book *Ren Zhai Zhi Zhi Fang Lun* 仁斋直指方论 (1264 AD).

The oral CHM formula *Ru xiang zhan luo san* 乳香盏落散, which contains pericarpium papaveris (罂粟壳) to treat unbearable headache, was introduced in the book published in the Yuan dynasty *Wei Sheng Bao Jian* 卫生宝鉴 (1283 AD). A book published in the Qing dynasty, *Wen Tang Ji Yan Fang* 文堂集验方 (1775 AD) described the symptoms and aetiology of *tou feng* 头风 in great detail and suggested taking a CHM formula orally as much as possible to reduce the symptoms. It is interesting to note that the ingredients (*bai zhi* 白芷 and *chuan xiong* 川芎, together with cow brain) were processed with alcohol and patients were suggested to take this formula as much as possible. Since this formula contained alcohol, when patients took it as much as possible and got drunk, they would fall asleep and their headaches would disappear the next day. This preparation was also named as *Huang niu nao zi jiu* 黄牛脑子酒, being documented in *Shou Shi Qing Bian* 寿世青编 (1667 AD) to treat long-term *pian zheng tou tong* 偏正头痛 (远年近日，偏正头痛). Therefore, taking alcohol and getting drunk to overcome migraine-like headache was considered as an effective method and was popular in the Qing dynasty (1645–1911 AD). It could be explained by the fact that being drunk itself could reduce a patient's sensations towards pain, and make patients easily fall asleep. After a whole night of sleep, the migraine symptom may have resolved automatically. Therefore, in the treatment of taking CHM together with alcohol, the alcohol may play a more important role than the CHM ingredients. In another book, *Lei Zheng Pu Ji Ben Shi Fang Shi Yi* 类证普济本事方释义 (1745 AD), it was suggested to sniff CHM *Tou ding san* 透顶散 into the nostril to treat long-term *tou feng* 头风 (不问年深日近).

In the Ming Guo period, an externally applying CHM method to treat long-term *pian tou feng* 偏头风 was recorded in *Fu Xi Mi Zhuan Jian Yan Fang* 鲔溪秘传简验方 (1918 AD): mix the powder of *she xiang* 麝香 and *zao jiao* 皂角, topically applying these powders on the headache area together with warm salt, using the combination of the herb's therapeutic effects and warmth to treat this disease.

Discussion of Chinese Herbal Medicine for Migraine

The frequently used oral CHM formulas and herbs identified from classical literature seem inconsistent compared to those recommended by contemporary literature (see Chapter 2). In current clinical practice, when applying oral CHM, the main syndromes to be considered are as follows:

- Liver *yang* uprising 肝阳上亢;
- Phlegm stagnation in the Orifices 痰浊蒙窍;
- Blood stasis in Orifices 瘀血阻窍;
- *Qi* and Blood deficiency 气血亏虚;
- Liver and Kidney *yin* deficiency 肝肾阴虚;
- Cold stagnated in the Liver meridian 寒凝肝脉.

Hence, the basic oral CHM formulas recommended, according to these syndromes, are *Tian ma gou teng yin* 天麻钩藤饮, *Ban xia bai zhu tian ma tang* 半夏白术天麻汤, *Tong qiao huo xue tang* 通窍活血汤, *Ba zhen tang* 八珍汤, *Qi ju di huang wan* 杞菊地黄丸 and *Wu zhu yu tang* 吴茱萸汤.

Our evaluation of classical literature showed that, in history, migraine was caused by both external pathogens (wind, cold, fire and heat) and internal pathogens (phlegm and *qi*), with wind invasion being the leading factor. Therefore, oral CHM formulas which aimed to expel wind were identified as the most frequent, such as *Qing kong gao* 清空膏, *Zhui feng san* 追风散 and *Cha tiao san* 茶调散.

Consequently, herbs that carry the function of expelling wind were shown in the herb frequency lists. On the other hand, in contemporary clinical practice, migraine is considered to be mainly caused by internal pathogens. Therefore, there are inconsistencies between the findings of classical literature and contemporary literature in terms of the oral CHM treatments.

In addition, some CHM formulas were used externally to treat this condition, including sniffing the CHM powders or inserting CHM suppositories into the nostrils (e.g. *Tou ding san* 透顶散, *Tong ding san* 通顶散 and *Long xiang san* 龙香散), topically applying CHM cream on the headache area (e.g. mixture of *ru xiang* 乳香 and *bi ma zi* 蓖麻子), or steaming therapy (e.g. *Long xiang san* 龙香散). Such external applications are also recommended in contemporary literature; however, using different herbs.

It should be noted that some toxic herbs (*xi xin* 细辛, *fu zi* 附子 and *wu tou* 乌头) were frequently used in oral CHM formulas. These herbs are currently restricted in some countries due to their toxicity. This can be explained by the fact that the aetiology of migraine was considered as cold invasion, while herbs of *xi xin* 细辛, *fu zi* 附子 and *wu tou* 乌头 carry the function of warming and unblocking meridians. In fact, the toxicity of these herbs was noted in history and some efforts have been made to reduce the toxicity when making CHM decoctions containing these herbs. For example, *gan cao* 甘草, honey, or *lv dou* 绿豆 (mung bean) were often used in the formulas containing *xi xin* 细辛 or *fu zi* 附子/*wu tou* 乌头 for detoxification when they were used to treat migraine.

Ying su ke 罂粟壳, the shell of poppy seed (*Papaver somniferum* L.), was found as the chief ingredient of one of the most frequently used oral CHM formulas in the 'most likely' migraine pool (*Ru xiang zhan luo san* 乳香盏落散). It was said that the use of this formula can treat unbearable headache (one side or both sides) (治男子妇人偏正头疼不可忍, 大有神效), in the book *Wei Sheng Bao Jian* 卫生宝鉴 (1281 AD). In addition, there is the treatment of mixing opium with rice, which can then be taken as pills (named *Yi li jin dan* 一粒金丹) to treat *pian tou feng* 偏头风, together with an oral CHM formula *Chuan xiong tang* 川芎汤. However, this pill should be limited and not taken more than two times, as introduced in the book *Ben Cao Pin Hui Jing Yao* 本草品汇精要 (1505 AD) (每服一丸, 未效再进, 不可多服).

The planting of poppy in China started from the Tang dynasty (618–907 AD), and the application of *ying su ke* 罂粟壳 for medical use started from the Song dynasty (960–1279 AD), as recorded in the book *Kai Bao Ben Cao* 开宝本草 (973 AD). This herb can be taken orally for relieving severe pain, cough and diarrhoea. According to a famous CM master, *Zhu Dan Xi* 朱丹溪 (1281–1358 AD), the function and its addictive properties were noted as 'although *ying su ke* 罂粟壳 functions rapidly when used as a drug, it can make patient addictive, therefore it should not be used for large doses or long-term' (其止病之功虽急, 杀人如剑, 宜深戒之).

According to these descriptions, it is known that opium has been used as an oral herb for almost 1,000 years in China, with the harm being noted. Such practice is consistent with the history of the medical use of opium in Western countries.

Acupuncture and Related Therapies

The 312 citations describing acupuncture and related therapies were found in 65 books. *Pu Ji Fang zhen jiu* 普济方针灸 (1406 AD) was the book that yielded the largest number of citations (*n* = 52). Other books that identified more than 20 citations included *Zhen Jiu Ji Cheng* 针灸集成 (1874 AD) (*n* = 29), *Zhen Jiu Zi Sheng Jing* 针灸资生经 (1220 AD) (*n* = 23), *Zhen Jiu Ju Ying* 针灸聚英 (1529 AD) (*n* = 20) and *Zhen Jiu Da Cheng* 针灸大成 (1601 AD) (*n* = 20).

Frequency of Treatment Citations by Dynasty

The majority of the identified citations (*n* = 251; 80.4%) were published in the Ming dynasty (1369–1644 AD) and the Qing dynasty (1645–1911 AD) (Table 3.13), which was identical to CHM citations. Two citations were found in two Japanese books published in the Qing dynasty. The earliest citations were identified from *Zhen Jiu Jia Yi Jing* 针灸甲乙经 (282 AD). These citations were obtained by the search terms *tou tong* 头痛, *jue tou tong* 厥头痛 and *nao feng* 脑风. A

Table 3.13.   Dynastic Distribution of Treatment Citations

Dynasty	No. of Treatment Citations
Before Tang dynasty (before 618 AD)	6
Tang and 5 dynasties (618–960 AD)	1
Song and Jin dynasties (961–1271 AD)	31
Yuan dynasty (1272–1368 AD)	10
Ming dynasty (1369–1644 AD)	159
Qing dynasty (1645–1911 AD)	92
Ming Guo/Republic of China (1912–1949 AD)	11
Japan	2
Total	312

Table 3.14. Acupuncture Treatments in 'Possible' Migraine Citations

Acupuncture Treatment	No. of Citations (*n*)
Acupuncture	73
Acupuncture and moxibustion	59
Moxibustion	38

couple of acupuncture points and meridians were introduced in this book with acupuncture therapy. The most recent citations were found in the book *Jin Zhen Mi Zhuan* 金针秘传, published in 1937 AD in the Ming Guo period. Several acupuncture points were described to treat this disease with acupuncture or/and moxibustion therapy.

Treatment with Acupuncture and Related Therapies

Of the 312 acupuncture and related therapies citations, 145 citations described acupuncture points or meridians for managing migraine without specifying treatment methods. A total of 73 (23.4%) citations stated acupuncture for therapy, while others mentioned moxibustion, alone or in combination with acupuncture therapy (Table 3.14).

Acupuncture points and meridians were obtained from all these citations for further analysis.

Most Frequent Acupuncture Points and Meridians in 'Possible' Migraine Citations

A total of 84 acupuncture points were found in the 'possible' migraine citations. The most frequently cited acupuncture points were from Governing meridian 督脉 (GV20 *Baihui* 百会, GV23 *Shangxing* 上星, GV21 *Qianding* 前顶, GV22 *Xinhui* 囟会, GV24 *Shenting* 神庭 and GV19 *Houding* 后顶), Bladder meridian (BL9 *Yuzhen* 玉枕, BL2 *Cuanzhu* 攒竹, BL62 *Shenmai* 申脉, BL63 *Jinmen* 金门 and BL10 *Tianzhu* 天柱) and Gallbladder meridian (GB19 *Naokong* 脑空, GB20 *Fengchi* 风池 and GB4 *Hanyan* 颔厌) (Table 3.15). Most of the frequently used acupuncture points were located on the head and neck

Table 3.15. Most Frequent Acupuncture Points in 'Possible' Migraine Citations

Acupuncture Point	No. of Citations (*n*)
TE23 *Sizhukong* 丝竹空	35
LU7 *Lieque* 列缺	33
LI4 *Hegu* 合谷	33
GB20 *Fengchi* 风池	33
GV20 *Baihui* 百会	23
GV23 *Shangxing* 上星	24
GB19 *Naokong* 脑空	21
GV21 *Qianding* 前顶	14
BL9 *Yuzhen* 玉枕	14
GB4 *Hanyan* 颔厌	13
GV22 *Xinhui* 囟会	11
BL2 *Cuanzhu* 攒竹	11
BL62 *Shenmai* 申脉	11
GV24 *Shenting* 神庭	11

(Continued)

Table 3.15.　(Continued)

Acupuncture Point	No. of Citations (*n*)
ST41 *Jiexi* 解溪	11
ST8 *Touwei* 头维	10
BL63 *Jinmen* 金门	9
GV19 *Houding* 后顶	8
SP2 *Dadu* 大都	8
BL10 *Tianzhu* 天柱	8
LU9 *Taiyuan* 太渊	8
LI11 *Quchi* 曲池	7
GB12 *Wangu* 完骨	7
HT3 *Shaohai* 少海	7

Table 3.16.　Most Frequent Meridians in 'Possible' Migraine Citations

Meridians	No. of Citations (*n*)
Gallbladder meridian	20
Triple Energisers meridian	20
Stomach meridian	20
Large Intestine meridian	19
Bladder meridian	5

region. This might indicate that the selection of these points was based on the local and nearby therapeutic effect of acupuncture points.

Ninety citations mentioned the meridians for treatment without specifying the acupuncture points. The most frequently described meridians included Gallbladder meridian (*n* = 20), Triple Energisers meridian (also known as *San jiao* 三焦 meridian) (*n* = 20), Stomach meridian (*n* = 20), Large Intestine meridian (*n* = 19) and Bladder meridian (*n* = 5) (Table 3.16). This reflects the clinical practice of selecting points from certain meridians to solve headaches which occur in those areas dominated by these meridians. This theory is consistent with the management of headaches in current clinical practice.

According to this approach, clinicians should firstly determine the diseased meridians, then select points from these meridians by taking the points' specific functions into consideration.

Most Frequent Acupuncture Points in 'Mostly Likely' Migraine Citations

Ten citations that mentioned acupuncture and related therapies were judged to be 'most likely' migraine citations. A total of 13 acupuncture points were extracted from these citations. Four acupuncture points were found in multiple citations: GB8 *Shuaigu* 率谷 (*n* = 3), ST8 *Touwei* 头维 (*n* = 2), GB13 *Benshen* 本神 (*n* = 2) and GB20 *Fengchi* 风池 (*n* = 2). All these points are located on the head or neck, reflecting the practice of using local points to treat headaches.

Discussion of Acupuncture for Migraine

A relatively small number of acupuncture citations were included in our evaluation. Although acupuncture-related therapies are frequently used to treat pain conditions, including headache (migraine), these treatments were commonly recorded in classical literature from the angle of introducing specific points' functions with their location and application, but without details of syndrome differentiation or symptoms being attached. Therefore, only a small number of acupuncture citations were included in the 'most likely' migraine citations pool since our screening criteria were based on the symptoms described by the citations.

Blood-letting therapy was used historically for migraine, but it is not considered a safe and hygienic method in clinical practice now. Through points frequency analysis, it was found that most of the points are located at the pain area including the head and neck. It should be noted that, since migraine-like conditions can be classified as headache caused by disease due to the blockage of certain meridians according to the location of pain, the meridian differentiation method was often used when selecting points for acupuncture. In such citations, details of acupuncture points may have not been stated and when selecting meridians for treatment, points may not be limited to those located in the pain area.

Other Therapies

A total of 19 citations introduced *Daoyin* 导引 exercise (body and mind exercise related to *qigong* 气功), lifestyle and diet self-management for treating migraine. The earliest citations of *Daoyin* 导引 exercise were found in the book *Zhu Bing Yuan Hou Lun* 诸病源候论 published in the Sui dynasty (610 AD). In the book chapter of *Yang Sheng Fang•Daoyin Fa* 养生方•导引法, it was suggested that if a person suffered from *tou feng* 头风, he should practise certain breathing exercise when seated, together with body stretching, and gentle massage on the head. By practising these exercises, the symptoms of *tou feng* 头风 may be relieved, hence patients' sleeping quality would be improved. Such therapy was continually used until the Qing dynasty (1645–1911 AD). For example, one citation identified from a book published in the Qing dynasty, *Dong Gong An Mo Mi Jue* 动功按摩秘诀, introduced details of daily body exercise in combination with diet and emotion control for the management of *tou tong* 头痛 (headache).

Classical Literature in Perspective

Migraine, known as *pian tou tong* 偏头痛 in the Chinese language in current clinical practice, is a type of severe headache characterised with specific symptoms. In history, migraine-like headaches have been described under different disease names. The earliest seen disease names were *shou feng* 首风 and *nao feng* 脑风 which were recorded in *Su Wen* 素问; then *tou feng* 头风 appeared in the book *Jin gui yao lue fang lun* 金贵要略方论 (219 AD). However, these diseases often referred to some headaches caused by external wind invasion or associated with other symptoms which are not related to migraine. The disease *pian tou tong* 偏头痛, was first seen in the book *Dong Yuan Shi Shu* 东垣十书 (1529 AD) published in the Ming dynasty (1369–1644 AD), which defined headache occurring on one side of the head. Along with the development of the understanding of this disease, more and more details corresponding to migraine in modern medicine were recorded in classical literature, for example, this disease is more prevalent in females than males, and it is accompanied with other symptoms such as change of sensations and sweating.

The aetiology of this disease from the CM point of view has evolved from external wind invasion to internal factors including Liver *qi* uprising, internal wind caused by Liver *yang* or Blood deficiency, Blood deficiency and stasis, phlegm and fire. When the combination of internal and external pathogens attacks the *Shao yang* 少阳, *Yang ming* 阳明 and Foot *Jue yin* 厥阴 meridians, headaches will occur and affect the corresponding areas of these meridians. Therefore, the treatments of this disease should take the CM syndrome differentiation from both angles into consideration, with CHM to focus on the external wind invasion and other internal factors and acupuncture treatment to focus on the affected meridians.

In current clinical practice, the treatment of acute migraine and prevention of the attacks of episodic migraine are both important for the management of this condition. However, our comprehensive evaluation of classical literature did not identify a clear differentiation of acute treatment and prevention treatment. This could be explained as, on one hand, the treatment principle of addressing external pathogens together with the underlying internal factors itself could be effective for preventing the recurrence of migraine attacks; and on the other hand, due to the limitation in understanding of migraine's pathological process, clinicians may have not paid enough attention to the prevention treatment of migraine.

It is noted that alcohol was considered effective in the management of acute migraine-like conditions. In fact, if a person who is suffering a migraine attack drinks alcohol and falls asleep, he/she may not feel the pain as much as being awake. After a whole night sleeping, the migraine headache may have reduced by itself.

However, overdrinking alcohol may cause other consequences; therefore, such method is not recommended as a treatment for migraine in current clinical practice. Furthermore, some herbs identified from classical literature as the treatment of migraine-like conditions should be used with caution in current practice, such as *ying su ke* 罂粟壳, *xi xin* 细辛, *fu zi* 附子 and *wu tou* 乌头 due to their addictive nature or toxicity, and some (e.g. *she xiang* 麝香) may be restricted under the Convention on International Trade in Endangered Species of Wild Fauna and Flora (CITES). Readers are advised to comply with relevant regulations.

References

1. Ma KW. (2000) Acupuncture: Its place in the history of Chinese medicine. *Acupunct Med* **18(2):** 88–99.

2. White A, Ernst E. (2004) A brief history of acupuncture. *Rheumatology (Oxford)* **43(5):** 662–663.

3. May BH, Lu Y, Lu C, *et al.* (2013) Systematic assessment of the representativeness of published collections of the traditional literature on Chinese medicine. *J Altern Complement Med* **19(5):** 403–409.

4. May BH, Lu C, Xue CC. (2012) Collections of traditional Chinese medical literature as resources for systematic searches. *J Altern Complement Med* **18(12):** 1101–1107.

5. Jia Hong Science and Technology Development Co. Ltd. (2014) *Zhong Hua Yi Dian* 中华医典 [*Encyclopaedia of Traditional Chinese Medicine,* 5th ed.] Hunan Electronic and Audio-Visual Publishing House, Changsha.

6. Tepper SJ, Tepper DE. (2014) *The Cleveland Clinic Manual of Headache Therapy.* Springer, New York.

7. 黄培新, 黄燕. (2013) 专科专病中医临床诊疗丛书 — 神经科专病中医临床诊治. 北京: 人民卫生出版社.

8. 孙怡. (2011) 实用中西医结合神经病学. 北京: 人民卫生出版社.

9. 赖新生. (2006) 针灸脑病学. 北京: 人民卫生出版社.

10. 王永炎, 张伯礼. (2007) 中医脑病学. 北京: 人民卫生出版社.

11. 曹克刚, 高颖. (2011) 中医内科常见病诊疗指南 (西医疾病部分) 偏头痛. 中国中医药现代远程教育. 北京: 中国中医药出版社.

12. 中国针灸学会. (2014) 循证针灸临床实践指南. 北京: 中国中医药出版社.

13. 秦旭华，唐怡，李祖伦. (2010) 中医对偏头痛认识沿革的探析. 中药与临床. **4:** 43–45.
14. 吴玉斌. 论头风病源流. (2014) 辽宁中医药大学学报 **1:** 136–137.
15. 黎婉玲. (2012) 偏头痛患者的中医体质特征研究 (Thesis). 南方医科大学.
16. 谢炜，史国军. (2011) 中药与西药对照治疗偏头痛的 Meta 分析. 热带医学杂志 **11(3):** 264–267.
17. 叶德宝. (2005) 偏头痛在中西医病名方面的探讨. 浙江中医学院学报 **29(6):** 9–10.
18. 王文静. (2017) 基于古今医案数据分析的偏头痛病证治规律研究 (Thesis). 广州中医药大学.
19. 赵凌，任玉兰，梁繁荣. (2009) 基于数据挖掘技术分析历代针灸治疗偏头痛的用穴特点. 中国针灸 **6:** 467–472.
20. 滕飞，杨宇峰，石岩. (2017) 头痛的中医诊疗理论框架. 中华中医药学刊 **35(9):** 2271–2273.
21. 吴银玲. (2010) 近年来中医治疗偏头痛综述. 湖北中医杂志 **32(11):** 80.

4

Methods for Evaluating Clinical Evidence

OVERVIEW

This chapter describes the methods used to identify and evaluate a range of Chinese medicine interventions for migraine in clinical studies. Studies identified through a comprehensive search were assessed against eligibility criteria. A review of the methodological quality of the studies was undertaken using standardised methods. Results from included studies were evaluated to provide an estimate of the effects of a range of Chinese medicine therapies.

Introduction

The use of Chinese medicine (CM) for migraine has been well described in the contemporary literature (see Chapter 2) and in classical CM (see Chapter 3). The evidence of CM therapies from modern literature will be presented in subsequent chapters. This chapter describes the methods used to evaluate clinical studies. Studies were evaluated following methods of the Cochrane Handbook of Systematic Reviews.[1] Interventions have been categorised as follows:

- Chinese herbal medicine (CHM) (Chapter 5)
- Acupuncture and other Chinese medicine therapies (Chapter 7)
- CM combination therapies (Chapter 8).

References to clinical trials were obtained and assessed by an expert group. Randomised controlled trials (RCTs), non-randomised controlled clinical trials (CCTs), and non-controlled studies were evaluated in detail. Non-randomised controlled clinical trials were evaluated using the same approach as RCTs, and have been described separately. Evidence from non-controlled studies is more difficult to evaluate; therefore the approach was taken to describe the characteristics of the study, details of the intervention and any adverse events. References to included studies are indicated by a letter followed by a number. Studies of CHM are indicated by an 'H' e.g. H1; studies of acupuncture and other Chinese medicine therapies are indicated by an 'A' e.g. A1; and studies of CM combination therapies indicated by a 'C' e.g. C1.

Search Strategy

Evidence was searched in English- and Chinese-language databases and the methods followed the Cochrane Handbook of Systematic Reviews.[1] English-language databases included PubMed; Excerpta Medica Database (Embase); Cumulative Index of Nursing and Allied Health Literature (CINAHL); Cochrane Central Register of Controlled Trials (CENTRAL), including the Cochrane Library, and Allied and Complementary Medicine Database (AMED); and Chinese-language databases including China BioMedical Literature (CBM), China National Knowledge Infrastructure (CNKI), Chongqing VIP (CQVIP) and Wanfang. Databases were searched from inception to March 2018. No restrictions were applied. Search terms were mapped to controlled vocabulary (where applicable), in addition to being searched as keywords.

To conduct a comprehensive search of the literature, searches were run according to the study design (reviews, controlled trials, non-controlled studies). This was done for each of the three intervention types (CHM, acupuncture and related therapies, and other CM therapies) resulting in nine searches in each of the nine databases:

1. CHM reviews;
2. CHM controlled trials (randomised and non-randomised);
3. CHM non-controlled studies;
4. Acupuncture-related therapies reviews;
5. Acupuncture-related therapies, controlled trials (randomised and non-randomised);

6. Acupuncture-related therapies non-controlled studies;
7. Other CM therapies reviews;
8. Other CM therapies, controlled trials (randomised and non-randomised);
9. Other CM therapies non-controlled studies.

Studies of combination CM therapies were identified through the above searches. In addition to electronic databases, reference lists of systematic reviews and included studies were searched for additional publications. Clinical trial registries were searched to identify clinical trials which were ongoing or completed, and where required, trial investigators were contacted to obtain data. The searched trial registries included the Australian New Zealand Clinical Trial Registry (ANZCTR), the Chinese Clinical Trial Registry (ChiCTR), the European Union Clinical Trials Register (EU-CTR) and the United States of America National Institutes of Health register (ClinicalTrials.gov).

Inclusion Criteria

- Study type: Controlled prospective studies with, or without, randomisation and uncontrolled studies (cohort, case series and case studies);
- Participants: Adults (aged between 18 years and 70 years) who were diagnosed with episodic migraine with, or without, aura according to clinical guidelines;[2–5]
- Interventions: Chinese herbal medicine, acupuncture and related therapies, or other CM therapies, alone or in combination with other CM therapies or with pharmacotherapy (Table 4.1). Studies combining CM therapies with pharmacotherapy/routine care were required to use the same pharmacotherapy/routine care in both the intervention and comparator groups;
- Comparators: Placebo, no treatment or waiting list, pharmacotherapies or other routine care therapies that are recommended in clinical practice guidelines;[2–5]
- Outcome measures: Studies that reported at least one of the pre-specified outcome measures (Table 4.2).

Table 4.1. Chinese Medicine Interventions Included in Clinical Evidence Evaluation

Category	Intervention
Chinese herbal medicines (CHM)	Oral CHM
Acupuncture-related and other Chinese medicine therapies	Acupuncture, acupressure and ear acupuncture
Combination Chinese medicine therapies	Combination therapies are defined as two or more Chinese medicine interventions from different categories administered together, e.g. CHM plus acupuncture, acupuncture plus *tuina* 推拿 therapy, acupuncture plus cupping therapy, etc.

Table 4.2. Pre-specified Outcomes

Outcome Categories	Acute Treatment or Preventive Treatment	Outcome Measures	Scoring
Pain-free at two hours	Acute	Percentage of study participants who were free of pain at two hours after treatment	Higher is better
Sustained pain freedom	Acute	Percentage of study participants who were free of pain at two hours and were also pain-free at 24 hours or 48 hours after treatment	Higher is better
Pain relief (from severe/moderate to mild or no pain) of acute migraine	Acute	Percentage of study participants who achieved pain relief	Higher is better
Migraine-associated symptoms	Acute	Nausea, vomiting, photophobia and phonophobia	Lower is better
Migraine frequency	Preventive	Frequency of migraine episodes	Lower is better
Number of migraine days	Preventive	Days of migraine with moderate or severe intensity	Lower is better

Table 4.2. (***Continued***)

Outcome Categories	Acute Treatment or Preventive Treatment	Outcome Measures	Scoring
Intensity of headache	Acute and preventive	Categorical rating scale	
Pain severity	Acute and preventive	VAS, NRS	0 to 10, or 0 to 100; lower is better
Responder rate	Preventive	Percentage of study participants who achieved a 50% reduction based on number of migraine days with moderate or severe intensity and migraine frequency	Higher is better
Duration of migraine attacks	Preventive	Duration of pain (in hours)	Lower is better
Acute medication usage	Preventive	—	Lower is better
Health-related quality of life	Preventive	MIDAS, HIT-6, MSQ	MIDAS, HIT-6: lower is better; MSQ: higher is better
Adverse events	Acute and preventive	Number and type of adverse events	

Abbreviations: HIT-6, Headache Impact Test-6; MIDAS, Migraine Disability Assessment; MSQ, Migraine Specific Quality of Life Questionnaire; NRS, numerical rating scale; VAS, visual analogue scale/score.

Exclusion Criteria

- Study type: Epidemiological studies, studies that compared CM therapy to other CM therapies; duplicated studies that reported same results: those published later were excluded;
- Participants: Patients aged less than 18 years or more than 70 years of age; menstrual-related migraine; chronic migraine (headache

occurring on 15 or more days per month for more than three months, which has the features of migraine headache on at least eight days per month);

- Intervention: Chinese medicine interventions not commonly practised worldwide;
- Comparators: Therapies not recommended by international clinical guidelines;
- Outcomes: Studies that did not report one of the predefined outcomes or reported the outcomes with different measures (e.g. effective rate not based on 50% of symptom relief).

Outcomes

Outcome measures were selected based on clinical guidelines,[4–8] review and discussion articles related to migraine clinical trial designs,[9–11] recently published systematic reviews[12–14] and high-quality RCTs.[15–20]

Since there is not any objective or laboratory test for migraine's severity, it was suggested that in clinical studies of migraine, the main outcome measures related to migraine symptoms should be based on information collected from a headache diary which captures the key assessment measures for clinical studies.[10,11] Also, the outcomes used to evaluate the effects of prevention treatment for episodic migraine and treatment for acute migraine attacks should focus on different aspects. Migraine-related quality of life (QoL) data should be collected from QoL questionnaires including Migraine Disability Assessment (MIDAS), Headache Impact Test-6 (HIT-6) and Migraine Specific Quality of Life Questionnaire (MSQ). Details are listed below.

Outcomes for Acute Migraine Treatment

The goals of acute (or symptomatic) migraine therapy are to relieve pain and the associated symptoms of migraine (e.g. nausea, vomiting, photophobia and phonophobia) rapidly and consistently, with minimal or no adverse events, and to relieve migraine-related disability so that the patient can return quickly to normal functioning.[4,5,7–9]

Primary Outcome Measures

- Pain-free at two hours after treatment, calculated as percentage of patients who were pain-free (at two hours after treatment);[4,5,7,9,10]
- Sustained pain freedom, defined as the percentage of study participants who are pain-free at two hours with no use of rescue medication or relapse (recurrence) within the subsequent 22[4,5,7–9] or 46 hours;[10]
- Pain relief or headache relief, defined as severe/moderate pain reduced to mild or no pain;[4,5,7–10]
- Responder rate, calculated as the percentage of study participants who achieved any of the above three outcomes.

Secondary Outcome Measures

Intensity of Headache

A categorical rating scale should be used to rate each headache's intensity as 0 = no pain, 1 = mild headache, 2 = moderate headache, and 3 = severe headache. Intensity alone is not recommended as a primary outcome measure. Intensity of headache is integrated into the primary outcome measure of number of headache days with moderate or severe intensity. Depending on the trial design, participants should be instructed to record the maximum intensity for each headache day/episode and/or each calendar day.[7,10]

Pain Severity: Visual Analogue Scale

Visual analogue scale (VAS) is a continuous measurement instrument[21] for subjective characteristics or attitudes that cannot be directly measured, such as pain intensity. It was described in 1921 for the first time.[22] A VAS consists of a line and two anchors (0 and 10 for pain), one at each end. When responding to a VAS item, respondents specify their level of pain by indicating a position along the continuous line between two endpoints.[23] The VAS provides researchers with a number of advantages. In comparison with discrete scales, measurement by a VAS is more exact and the scale needs less explanation for research participants. With the spread of computerisation nowadays, reading data from a VAS is much easier.

Numeric Rating Scale

Numeric rating scale (NRS), designed by Budzynski and Melzack, is another widely used measurement instrument to verify pain intensity. Like a VAS, there are also two points on each end of a horizontal line, marked as zero to 10, or zero to 100, but the line is separated into 11 or 101 parts equally by numbers and the responders point out a number to represent their pain intensity. Meanwhile as the number goes bigger, the pain intensity gets larger.[24] In comparison, the line is empty in a VAS, which can be more accurate.

Migraine-associated Symptoms

The presence or absence of migraine-associated symptoms including nausea, photophobia and phonophobia can be assessed at two hours after treatment.[7,10] The severity of each of these symptoms can also be recorded as 0 = none, 1 = mild, 2 = moderate, and 3 = severe.[7,10]

Outcomes for Prevention Treatment of Episodic Migraine

Prevention therapy should be considered when migraine has a substantial impact despite use of acute medications, or when high attack frequency puts patients at risk for medication overuse headache.[6,8] The purpose of prevention treatment is to reduce the frequency and severity of migraine attacks.[8] A prophylactic therapy is usually considered effective if the patient's migraine attack frequency, or the number of days with headache per month, is reduced by 50% or more,[6,10] or 30–50%.[8] In addition, a reduction in headache intensity and migraine-related disability can also be considered to assess the effectiveness of prophylactic therapy.[6,10]

Primary Outcome Measures

- Number of migraine attacks per evaluation interval (four weeks or one month).[4–6,8–10] A migraine attack that is interrupted by sleep, or temporarily remits, and then recurs within 48 hours should be recorded as one attack and not two. An attack treated successfully with medication but with relapse within 48 hours should be considered one attack.
- Number of migraine days per evaluation interval (four weeks or one month).[6,10] A migraine day is defined as a day with migraine (meets the criteria of migraine without aura, migraine with aura, or probable migraine defined in the International Classification of Headache Disorders (ICHD), 3rd ed.).[11] To record a migraine day, participants must:

  o Have a day with headache of four hours duration;
  o Meet the criteria of migraine without aura, migraine with aura, or probable migraine defined in the ICHD-3;[2] or
  o Take medication of triptan or ergot with headache relief within two hours.

  Migraine days are easier to record in headache diaries and may be very useful in large-scale, long-term, pragmatic trials. However, migraine days, unlike migraine attacks, represent a composite endpoint because it incorporates attack duration. It can be argued that the efficacy endpoint 'migraine days' is not as accurate (neither as sensitive nor as specific) as 'migraine attacks' when the primary study objective is the evaluation of a preventative agent.[10]

Secondary Outcome Measures

- Responder rate. Responder rates should be defined as a 30–50% reduction based on (1) headache days with moderate or severe intensity; (2) migraine days; or (3) migraine episodes compared with the baseline period.[8,10]

  Another type of effective rate is the most commonly used outcome measure in clinical trials conducted in China.[25,26] This is calculated as the percentage of participants who achieved certain improvement (based on a variety of symptoms). The cut-off line of 'effective' also varied across different guidelines or studies. Since most of clinical evidence is collected from the studies conducted in China, this type of effective rate is the most frequently used one among the studies included in our evaluation. In order to capture the treatment effects measured by this outcome in a consistent manner with worldwide accepted approach, we selected the effective rate calculated based on a 50% of reduction and merged these data under responder rate.

- Duration of migraine in hours. Participants may record the start and stop time of each headache episode. Duration alone is not recommended as an outcome measure, since the duration of migraine may be modified by acute treatment, and the start and stop times of migraine cannot be determined with certainty due to participants' different sleep behaviour or different tolerability.[10,11]
- Intensity of headache (see above).
- Pain severity, including VAS or NRS (see above).
- Acute treatment utilisation.

Change in acute medication use is an important secondary outcome because it may reflect a change in headache status.[10]

Health Care Outcomes/Quality of Life

Migraine patients' health-related quality of life can be evaluated by the general quality of life questionnaire (e.g. SF-36) or disease-specific health-related quality of life and disability instruments, with the MIDAS being the most commonly used one. Others such as HIT-6 and MSQ are also commonly used in migraine clinical trials.

Migraine Disability Assessment Test

MIDAS is a questionnaire to determine how severely migraines affect patients' quality of life. It was developed to assess headache-related disability with the aim of improving migraine care.[4,27] The

MIDAS score was also correlated with physicians' assessments of need for medical care. From studies completed to date, the MIDAS questionnaire has been shown to be internally consistent, highly reliable and valid, and it correlates with physicians' clinical judgment. These features support its suitability for use in clinical practice.[27]

In the MIDAS questionnaire, patients are asked questions about the frequency and duration of their headaches, as well as how often these headaches limited their ability to participate in activities at work, at school or at home.

The questionnaire contains questions like the ones below:

1. On how many days in the last three months did you miss work or school because of your headaches?
2. How many days in the last three months was your productivity at work or school reduced by half or more because of your headaches? (Do not include days you counted in question 1 where you missed work or school.)
3. On how many days in the last three months did you not do household work (such as housework, home repairs and maintenance, shopping, and caring for children and relatives) because of your headaches?
4. How many days in the last three months was your productivity in household work reduced by half or more because of your headaches? (Do not include days you counted in question 3 where you did not do household work.)
5. On how many days in the last three months did you miss family, social or leisure activities because of your headaches?

The patient's score consists of the total of these five questions.

Additionally, there is a section for patients to share with their doctors answers to questions like the ones below:

- On how many days in the last three months did you have a headache? (If a headache lasted more than one day, count each day.)
- On a scale of 0 to 10, on average how painful were these headaches? (where 0 = no pain at all and 10 = pain as bad as it can be).

Once scored, the test gives the patient an idea of how debilitating his/her migraines are based on this scale:

- 0 to 5: MIDAS Grade I, little or no disability;
- 6 to 10: MIDAS Grade II, mild disability;
- 11 to 20: MIDAS Grade III, moderate disability;
- 21+: MIDAS Grade IV, severe disability.

Headache Impact Test-6

The HIT-6 is a brief tool for assessing the impact of headache in both clinical research and practice.[4,28] The development and validation study indicated that the HIT-6 possessed good psychometric properties among headache sufferers.[29] It is recognised worldwide that HIT-6 is a highly reliable and internally consistent, and it has been translated into several languages.

The HIT-6 consists of six items: pain, social functioning, role functioning, vitality, cognitive functioning and psychological distress.[29] The HIT-6 can be useful for assessing headache-related disability over a one-month time period.[30] The patient answers each of the six related questions using one of the following five responses: 'never', 'rarely', 'sometimes', 'very often' or 'always'. These responses are summed to produce a total HIT-6 score that ranges from 36 to 78, where a higher score indicates a greater impact of headache on the daily life of the respondent. Scores can be interpreted using four groupings that indicate the severity of headache/migraine impact on the migraine patient's life.[29]

The HIT-6 questionnaire contains questions like the following:

1. When you have headaches, how often is the pain severe? (never, rarely, sometimes, very often, always)
2. How often do headaches limit your ability to do usual daily activities including household work, work, school or social activities?
3. When you have a headache, how often do you wish you could lie down?
4. In the past four weeks, how often have you felt too tired to do work or daily activities because of your headaches?

5. In the past four weeks, how often have you felt fed-up or irritated because of your headaches?
6. In the past four weeks, how often did headaches limit your ability to concentrate on work or daily activities?

Migraine Specific Quality of Life Questionnaire

The MSQ contains 14 items and was developed to assess the effects of migraine and its treatment on patients' health-related quality of life.[31] The MSQ was designed to measure three meaningful dimensions:

1. Role Function-Restrictive (seven questions): Examines the degree to which performance of daily activities is limited by migraine;
2. Role Function-Preventive (four questions): Examines the degree to which performance of daily activities is prevented by migraine;
3. Emotional Function (three questions): Examines feelings of frustration and helplessness due to migraine.

Through validity and reliability studies,[32] it was confirmed that the MSQ is a reliable instrument in the assessment of quality of life for patients with migraine with items that can be summed without weights, and the MSQ has demonstrated evidence of construct validity.[32]

Adverse Event

Data of adverse events were also collected and pooled for analyses where possible to provide evidence of safety of the CM therapies.

Given that all the above listed outcome endpoints are the most commonly reported outcomes in previous clinical studies, they were selected in our systematic evaluation of clinical evidence in the subsequent chapters where possible.

Risk of Bias Assessment

Risk of bias was assessed for RCIs using the Cochrane Collaboration's tool.[1] In clinical trials, bias can be categorised as selection bias, performance bias, detection bias, attrition bias and reporting bias. Each domain is assessed to determine whether the bias is at 'low', 'high' or 'unclear' risk. 'Low' risk of bias indicates that bias is unlikely, 'high' risk indicates plausible bias that seriously weakens confidence in the results and 'unclear' bias indicates lack of information or uncertainty over potential bias and raises some doubt about the results. Risk of bias assessment was verified by two people and disagreement was resolved by discussion or consultation with a third person.

Risk of bias is categorised using the following six domains:

- Sequence generation: The method used to generate the allocation sequence is given in sufficient detail to allow an assessment of whether it should produce comparable groups. A 'low' risk of bias refers to a random-number table or computer random generator. A 'high' risk of bias includes studies that describe a non-random sequence generation such as odd or even date of birth or date of admission.
- Allocation concealment: The method used to conceal the allocation sequence is given in enough detail to determine whether intervention allocations could have been foreseen before or during enrolment. A 'low' risk of bias includes central randomisation or sealed envelopes and 'high' risk of bias includes open random sequence or date of birth.
- Blinding of participants and personnel: Measures used to describe if the study participants and personnel are blind to the intervention received. In addition, information relating to whether the blinding was effective is also assessed. Studies that ensure blinding of participants and personnel are at 'low' risk of bias. If the study is not blind or incompletely blind, it is at 'high' risk of bias.
- Blinding of outcome assessors: Measures used to describe if the outcome assessors are blind to knowledge of which intervention a participant received. In addition, information relating to whether the blinding was effective is also assessed. Studies that ensure blinding of outcome assessors are at 'low' risk of bias. If the study is not blind, or incompletely blind, it is at 'high' risk of bias.

- Incomplete outcome data: Completeness of outcome data for each main outcome, including drop-outs, exclusions from the analysis with numbers missing in each group, and reasons for drop-out or exclusions. Studies with 'low' risk of bias would include all outcome data, or if there is missing data, it is unlikely to relate to the true outcome or is balanced between groups. Studies at 'high' risk of bias would have unexplained missing data and the difference in the proportion of incomplete outcome data across groups is of concern.
- Selective reporting: Selective outcome reporting has been defined as the selection of a subset of the original variables recorded for inclusion in publication of trials. Studies with a published protocol and which include all pre-specified outcomes in their report would be at 'low' risk of bias. Studies at 'high' risk of bias would not include all pre-specified outcomes or the outcome data may be reported incompletely.

Statistical Analyses

Frequency of CM syndromes, CHM formulas, herbs and acupuncture points reported in included studies are presented using descriptive statistics. Chinese medicine syndromes reported in two or more studies are presented. The ten most frequently reported CHM formulas and 20 most frequently reported herbs are presented and were used in at least two studies, although for CHM formulas this was not always possible. The top ten acupuncture points used in two or more studies are presented, or as available.

Definitions of statistical tests and results are described in the glossary. Dichotomous data are reported as a risk ratio (RR) with 95% confidence interval (CI), and continuous data are reported as mean difference (MD) or standard mean difference (SMD) with 95% CI. For dichotomous data, when the RR is greater than one and the upper and lower values of the 95% CI are both greater than one, this indicates we can be 95% certain that there is a difference between the groups and that the true effect lies within these CIs. The same is true for values less than one. In such cases, we say there is a 'significant difference' between the groups. For continuous data, when the MD is greater than zero and both the upper and lower values of the 95% CI are greater than zero, we say there is a 'significant difference' between the groups. The same is true on the negative side of the scale.[1]

For all analyses, RR, MD or SMD together with 95% CI were reported, together with a formal test for heterogeneity using the I^2 statistic. An I^2 score greater than 50% was considered to indicate substantial heterogeneity.[1] Where possible and appropriate, planned subgroup analyses included duration of disease or treatment, CM formula and comparator types. Available case analysis with a random effects model was used in all analyses. The random effects model was used to take into account the clinical heterogeneity likely to be encountered within and between included studies and the variation in treatment effects between included studies.

Assessment Using Grading of Recommendations Assessment, Development and Evaluation

The Grading of Recommendations Assessment, Development and Evaluation (GRADE) approach was used.[33] The GRADE approach summarises and rates the strength and certainty (quality) of evidence in systematic reviews using a structured process for presenting evidence summaries. The results are presented in summary-of-findings tables.[34] The results provide an important overview for migraine outcomes.

A panel of experts was established to evaluate the certainty of evidence. The panel included the systematic review team, CM practitioners, integrative medicine experts, research methodologists and conventional medicine physicians. The experts were asked to rate the clinical importance of key interventions from CHM, acupuncture therapies and other CM therapies, as well as comparators and outcomes. Results were collated and based on the rating scores and subsequent discussion, a consensus on the content for the summary-of-findings tables was achieved.

The certainty of evidence for each outcome was rated according to five factors outlined in the GRADE approach. The certainty of evidence may be rated based on:

- Limitations in study design (risk of bias);
- Inconsistency of results (unexplained heterogeneity);
- Indirectness of evidence (interventions, populations and outcomes important to the patients with the condition);
- Imprecision (uncertainty about the results);
- Publication bias (selective publication of studies).

These five factors are additive and a reduction in more than one factor will reduce the certainty of the evidence for that outcome. The GRADE approach also includes three domains that can be rated up, including large magnitude of an effect, dose-response gradient and effect of plausible residual confounding. However, these three domains relate to observational studies including cohort, case-control, before-after and time-series studies. The GRADE summaries in this book only include RCTs; therefore these three domains for rating up were not assessed.

Treatment recommendations can also be assessed using the GRADE approach, but due to the diverse nature of CM practice, treatment recommendations were not included with the summary of findings. Therefore the reader is able to interpret the evidence with reference to the local practice environment. It should also be noted that the GRADE approach requires judgments about the certainty of evidence and some subjective assessment. However, the experience of the panel members suggests the judgments are reliable and transparent representations of the certainty of evidence.

The GRADE levels of evidence are grouped into four categories:

1. 'High' certainty: We are very confident that the true effect lies close to that of the estimate of the effect;
2. 'Moderate' certainty: We are moderately confident in the effect estimate. The true effect is likely to be close to the estimate of the effect, but there is a possibility that it is substantially different;

3. 'Low' certainty: Our confidence in the effect estimate is limited. The true effect may be substantially different from the estimate of the effect;

4. 'Very low' certainty: We have very little confidence in the effect estimate. The true effect is likely to be substantially different from the estimate of effect.

References

1. Higgins J, Green S, (eds.) (2011) Cochrane Handbook for Systematic Reviews of Interventions Version 5.1.0. The Cochrane Collaboration. Available from: http://www.cochrane-handbook.org.

2. Headache Classification Committee of the International Headache Society (IHS). (2018) The International Classification of Headache Disorders, 3rd ed. *Cephalalgia* **38(1):** 1–211.

3. Headache Classification Subcommittee of the International Headache Society. (2004) The International Classification of Headache Disorders, 2nd ed. *Cephalalgia* **24(Suppl 1):** 9–160.

4. 李舜伟, 李焰生, 刘若卓, *et al.* (2011) 中国偏头痛诊断治疗指南. 中国疼痛医学杂志. *Chin J Pain Med* **17(2):** 65–86.

5. 中华医学会疼痛学分会头面痛学组, 中国医师协会神经内科医师分会疼痛和感觉障碍专委会. (2016) 中国偏头痛防治指南. 中国疼痛医学杂志 *Chin J Pain Med* **22(10):** 721–727.

6. Pringsheim T, Davenport W, Mackie G, *et al.*; Canadian Headache Society Prophylactic Guidelines Development Group. (2012) Canadian Headache Society guideline for migraine prophylaxis. *Can J Neurol Sci* **39(2 Suppl 2):** S1–S59.

7. Worthington I, Pringsheim T, Gawel MJ, *et al.*; Canadian Headache Society Acute Migraine Treatment Guideline Development Group. (2013) Canadian Headache Society guideline: Acute drug therapy for migraine headache. *Can J Neurol Sci* **40(5 Suppl 3):** S1–S80.

8. Scottish Intercollegiate Guidelines Network (SIGN). (2018) Pharmacological management of migraine (SIGN publication no. 155). Available from: http://www.sign.ac.uk.

9. 于生元, 陈敏. (2014) 成人偏头痛的药物治疗策略. 中国新药杂志. **23(14):** 1631–1636.

10. Tfelt-Hansen P, Pascual J, Ramadan N, *et al*; International Headache Society Clinical Trials Subcommittee. (2012) Guidelines for controlled trials of drugs in migraine, 3rd ed. A guide for investigators. *Cephalalgia* **32(1):** 6–38.

11. Tassorelli C, Diener HC, Dodick DW, *et al*; International Headache Society Clinical Trials Standing Committee. (2018) Guidelines of the International Headache Society for controlled trials of preventive treatment of chronic migraine in adults. *Cephalalgia* **38(5):** 815–832.

12. Meissner K, Fässler M, Rücker G, *et al.* (2013) Differential effectiveness of placebo treatments: A systematic review of migraine prophylaxis. *JAMA Intern Med* **173(21):** 1941–1951.

13. Linde K, Allais G, Brinkhaus B, *et al.* (2016) Acupuncture for the prevention of episodic migraine. *Cochrane Database Syst Rev* **6**: CD001218.

14. Yang Y, Que Q, Ye X, Zheng Gh (2016). Verum versus sham manual acupuncture for migraine: A systematic review of randomised controlled trials. *Acupunct Med* **34(2):** 76–83.

15. Alecrim-Andrade J, Maciel-Júnior JA, Carnè X, *et al.* (2008) Acupuncture in migraine prevention: A randomized sham controlled study with 6-months posttreatment follow-up. *Clin J Pain* **24(2):** 98–105.

16. Wang LP, Zhang XZ, Guo J, *et al.* (2011) Efficacy of acupuncture for migraine prophylaxis: A single-blinded, double-dummy, randomized controlled trial. *Pain* **152(8):** 1864–1871.

17. Li Y, Zheng H, Witt CM, *et al.* (2012) Acupuncture for migraine prophylaxis: A randomized controlled trial. *CMAJ* **104(4):** 401–410.

18. Foroughipour M, Golchian AR, Kalhor M, *et al.* (2014) A sham-controlled trial of acupuncture as an adjunct in migraine prophylaxis. *Acupunct Med* **32(1):** 12–16.

19. Zhao L, Liu J, Zhang F, *et al.* (2014) Effects of long-term acupuncture treatment on resting-state brain activity in migraine patients: A randomized controlled trial on active acupoints and inactive acupoints. *PLoS One* **9(6):** e99538.

20. Zhao L, Chen J, Li Y, *et al.* (2017) The long-term effect of acupuncture for migraine prophylaxis: A randomized clinical trial. *JAMA Intern Med* **177(4):** 508–515.

21. Flynn D, Schaik VP, Wersch AV. (2004) A comparison of multi-item Likert and visual analogue scales for the assessment of transactionally defined coping function. *Eur J Psychol Assess* **20(1):** 49–58.

22. Hayes MHS, Patterson DG. (1921) Experimental development of the graphics rating method. *Physiol Bull* **18:** 98–99.

23. Reips UD, Funke F. (2008) Interval-level measurement with visual analogue scales in Internet-based research: VAS generator. *Behav Res Methods* **40(3):** 699–704.

24. 宋文阁, 王春亭, 傅志俭. (2008) 实用临床疼痛学. 郑州: 河南科学技术出版社.

25. 孙增华, 杨玉金. (1995) 偏头痛诊断疗效评定标准意见. 中风与神经疾病杂志 **11(2):** 110.

26. 郑筱萸. (2002) 中药新药临床研究指导原则(试行). 中国医药科技出版社.

27. Stewart WF, Lipton RB, Dowson AJ, Sawyer J. (2001) Development and testing of the Migraine Disability Assessment (MIDAS) Questionnaire to assess headache-related disability. *Neurology* **56(6 Suppl 1):** S20–S28.

28. Rendas-Baum R, Yang M, Varon SF, *et al.* (2014) Validation of the Headache Impact Test (HIT-6) in patients with chronic migraine. *Health Qual Life Outcomes* **12:** 117.

29. Kosinski M, Bayliss MS, Bjorner JB, *et al.* (2003) A six-item short-form survey for measuring headache impact: the HIT-6. *Qual Life Res* **12(8):** 963–974.

30. Shin HE, Park JW, Kim YI, Lee KS. (2008) Headache Impact Test-6 (HIT-6) scores for migraine patients: Their relation to disability as measured from a headache diary. *J Clin Neurol* **4(4):** 158–163.

31. Jhingran P, Davis SM, LaVange LM, *et al.* (1998) MSQ: Migraine-Specific Quality-of-Life Questionnaire. Further investigation of the factor structure. *Pharmacoeconomics* **13(6):** 707–717.

32. Martin BC, Pathak DS, Sharfman MI, *et al.* (2000) Validity and reliability of the migraine-specific quality of life questionnaire (MSQ Version 2.1). *Headache* **40(3):** 204–215.

33. Schunemann H, Brozek J, Guyatt G, Oxman A, eds. (2013) GRADE handbook for grading quality of evidence and strength of recommendations. The GRADE Working Group. Available from: http: //www.guidelinedevelopment.org/handbook/.

5

Clinical Evidence for Chinese Herbal Medicine

OVERVIEW

This chapter evaluates the available Chinese herbal medicine clinical evidence for its effects and safety on migraine. Where appropriate, Chinese herbal medicine treatments are pooled in meta-analyses to assess their overall affects for different outcome measures. The certainty of evidence is also evaluated to assess the strength of available data. Frequently used Chinese herbal medicine formulas and herbs are summarised. Ten systematic reviews and 68 clinical studies were included in the evaluation. There is promising evidence supporting the use of oral CHM for preventing migraine.

Introduction

Chinese herbal medicine (CHM) has been examined by many clinical studies which have been published in scientific journals, both in China and internationally. A rigorous screening process was undertaken to identify clinical studies of CHM for the treatment of acute migraine, as well as migraine prevention therapies. These studies included randomised controlled trials (RCTs), non-randomised controlled clinical trials (CCTs) and non-controlled studies. Evidence from RCTs has been pooled for evaluation of the efficacy and safety of CHM alone, or in combination with conventional therapy for episodic migraine. Controlled clinical trials were evaluated using the same approach as for RCTs and these results are described separately. Evidence from non-controlled studies is more difficult to evaluate;

therefore the approach was taken to describe the characteristics of the study, details of the intervention and any adverse events (AEs). The findings of the literature search are presented in this chapter.

Previous Systematic Reviews

Our comprehensive search identified ten previously published systematic review articles that evaluated the effects of CHM for the prophylactic (preventive) treatment of migraine.

Shi (2011)[1] evaluated three widely used CHM formulas, namely *Chuan xiong cha tiao san* 川芎茶调散 (*n* = 7), *Yang xue qing nao ke li* 养血清脑颗粒 (*n* = 29) and *Xue fu zhu yu tang* 血府逐淤汤 (*n* = 16), using routine care or placebo as a comparator. The Jadad scale was used to assess the methodological quality of the included studies. Meta-analysis suggested that CHM was more effective than controls for responder rate, regardless of whether CHM was used as an add-on therapy. On the other hand, the CHM group seemed safer with less AEs reported; however, information of AEs was not reported by almost half of the included studies. The methodological quality of included RCTs was 'low' and the detected publication bias may indicate inaccurate effectiveness of CHM.

Xie (2011)[2] systematically reviewed the effectiveness and safety of oral CHMs, including herbal decoctions and manufactured CHM products. Twenty-three RCTs published in Chinese were included in the review. All included RCTs compared CHM to a pharmacotherapy recommended in guidelines, such as flunarizine and nimodipine. This review used the Jadad scale and the risk of bias tool of the Cochrane method for intervention[3] to assess the methodological quality of included studies. According to the analyses of this review, the authors found that a higher responder rate was achieved in the CHM group than the pharmacotherapy group. Due to the limitations of methodological quality and follow-up, the authors suggested that more rigorously designed RCTs are required to confirm the evidence of CHM.

Zeng (2013)[4] systematically reviewed the effectiveness and safety of an oral CHM product, *Tong xin luo jiao nang* 通心络胶囊. Ten

RCTs published in Chinese were included in this review, comparing *Tong xin luo jiao nang* 通心络胶囊 (with or without flunarizine) to flunarizine alone. Methodological quality of included RCTs was assessed using the Cochrane risk of bias tool. Meta-analysis of two RCTs showed that *Tong xin luo jiao nang* 通心络胶囊 was more effective than flunarizine for responder rate. In terms of AE, mild abdominal pain in the CHM group was observed in one RCT. Due to the limitations of methodological quality and lack of meta-analysis for other outcome measures recommended by clinical guidelines, the evidence provided by this review was not conclusive.

Tan (2014)[5] systematically reviewed the effectiveness and safety of *Tou tong ning* 头痛宁, one of the widely used CHM products. Four Chinese databases were searched with ten RCTs being included. Five RCTs compared *Tou tong ning* 头痛宁 to flunarizine and another five RCTs evaluated the add-on effects to flunarizine. The methodological quality of the included studies was evaluated using the Cochrane risk of bias assessment. Meta-analyses showed that the overall effect of CHM group was superior to the flunarizine group and the add-on effect of CHM to flunarizine was also significant. In addition, the CHM group reported less AEs than the flunarizine group. The poor methodological quality limited the certainty of evidence provided by this review and rigorous multi-centre RCTs were needed to confirm the evidence.

Chen (2014)[6] also systematically reviewed the effectiveness and safety of *Tou tong ning* 头痛宁. Twenty-seven RCTs published in Chinese were included in this review, comparing *Tou tong ning* 头痛宁 of various dosages with conventional Western medicine. Modified Jadad scale was applied to assess the quality of RCTs. Meta-analysis showed that *Tou tong ning* 头痛宁 was superior to Western medicine in terms of responder rate and was associated with less AEs. Limitations regarding methodological quality and lack of outcome measures prevented any conclusion to be drawn.

Xiao *et al.* (2015)[7] evaluated the efficacy and safety of five types of traditional Chinese patent medicines (TCPMs) compared to placebo in migraineurs. Seven RCTs, with a total of 582 migraine patients, were selected in the review. The methodological quality of the included studies was assessed with the risk of bias. According to the meta-analysis, TCPMs were more effective than placebo for reducing the frequency of migraine attacks, as well as headache intensity and improving the responder rate. The AEs of TCPMs were not different from those of placebo. The authors concluded that TCPMs could be recommended as an evidence-based pharmaco-therapy option for migraine. However, the CHM products and their herb ingredients varied across studies, making it unclear which TCPM is more effective than others, since subgroup analyses based on the CHM were not performed.

Wang (2016)[8] systematically reviewed the effectiveness and safety of *Du liang ruan jiao nang* 都梁软胶囊 for treating migraine without aura with a common Chinese medicine (CM) syndrome (Blood stasis in the brain) using the Western medicine flunarizine as comparator. This review included three RCTs published in Chinese. The methodological quality of included RCTs was assessed using the risk of bias tool of the Cochrane method for intervention. Compared to flunarizine, commonly used for episodic migraine prevention, meta-analysis of three RCTs suggested that *Du liang ruan jiao nang* 都梁软胶囊 was beneficial in increasing responder rate. However, except the one RCT that evaluated CHM for a 90-day duration, the other two studies applied CHM treatment for only 15 days, which is insufficient to detect the prophylactic effects for migraine. More importantly, these RCTs did not include a follow-up phase; therefore the long-term prophylactic effects of CHM could not be confirmed. Due to the limitations of including a small number of studies and lack of meta-analysis for other outcome measures recommended by clinical guidelines, the evidence provided by this review was not conclusive.

Lai (2017)[9] systematically reviewed CHM compared to flunarizine for the treatment of migraine. A total of 25 studies published in Chinese were included in this review. The quality assessment was conducted by two reviewers using the Cochrane risk of bias tool. According to the analyses, CHM could improve the responder rate; reduce the recurrence rate; and decrease headache intensity, frequency of migraine attacks, number of migraine days and duration of each migraine attack. In addition, the plasma viscosity was also reduced by CHM. However, the CHM formulas used by the included studies varied greatly and similar limitations were found in the included studies.

Yan (2017)[10] evaluated oral CHM for migraine of Liver *yang* uprising syndrome. Sixteen RCTs were included in the review. Jadad scale was used to assess the methodological quality. Fifteen studies compared CHM to routine care and one RCT compared CHM to placebo. Meta-analyses showed that the CHM group achieved a higher responder rate than the routine care group ($n = 13$) and CHM significantly reduced the frequency of migraine attacks compared to routine care ($n = 4$). In terms of AEs, few mild gastrointestinal symptoms were reported by the CHM group, but the number of occasions was lower than the AEs reported by the routine care group. This review also pointed out the limitations of poor methodological quality and lack of outcome measures.

Identification of Clinical Studies

A search of nine English and Chinese language databases identified 12,773 potentially relevant citations, of which 1,713 required full text retrieval to determine eligibility for inclusion (Fig. 5.1). After assessment against rigorous inclusion criteria, 66 clinical studies which evaluated oral CHM for migraine were included in our evaluation, including 62 RCTs (H1–H62), two CCTs (H64, H65) and three non-controlled studies (H66–H68). Controlled studies (RCTs and CCTs) were evaluated to assess the efficacy and safety of CHM for migraine prevention, and details from non-controlled study are described. Of all included studies, 66 studies assessed the effects of CHM for preventing episodic migraine, one study evaluated the effects of CHM for both acute migraine management and episodic migraine prevention (H30) and another one study (H63) only evaluated the effects of CHM for acute migraine management (Fig. 5.1).

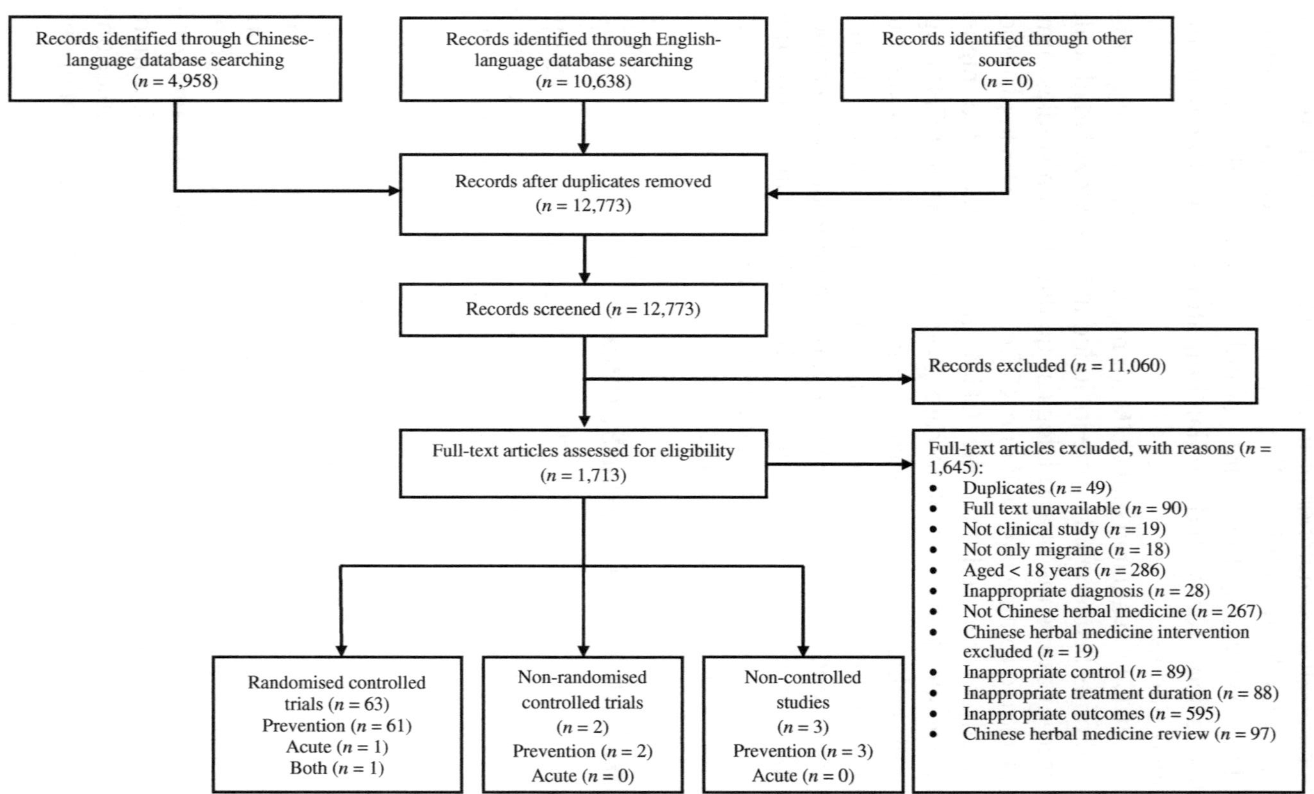

Fig. 5.1. Flowchart of study selection process: Chinese herbal medicine

Oral Chinese Herbal Medicine for Migraine Prevention

In total, 67 clinical studies assessed the effects of oral CHM for preventing episodic migraine, including 62 RCTs (H1–H62), two CCTs (H64, H65) and three non-controlled studies (H66–H68).

Randomised Controlled Trials of Oral Chinese Herbal Medicine

In total 62 RCTs investigated oral CHM (H1–H62). A total of 5,028 participants were included in these studies. Among the studies which provided information of participants' gender, there were more females than males (3,047 versus 1,749, respectively). The age of all patients included in these studies ranged from 18 years (H24) to 65 years of age (H26), with the average age being 39.19 years.

Of all included RCTs, ten studies (H1, H2, H7, H12, H25, H32, H37, H41, H59, H60) compared oral CHM to placebo (with, or without, pharmacotherapy as co-intervention in both groups); 37 studies compared oral CHM with pharmacotherapy and the other 15 studies (H4, H6, H9, H17, H27, H29–H31, H34, H40, H45, H49, H51, H53, H54) evaluated the add-on effects of oral CHM by comparing the combination of oral CHM with some forms of pharmacotherapy to the same pharmacotherapy alone. The efficacy of CHM was analysed and presented under each category of comparisons. The treatment duration ranged from 28 days (H54, H55, H57, H58, H60, H62) to 90 days (H13, H20, H21, H26, H32, H42) with the average treatment duration being 47 days.

Twenty-nine studies reported information of CM syndrome, with the most commonly seen syndrome being Blood stasis 瘀血阻滞 (*n* = 15) and Liver *yang* uprising 肝阳上亢 (*n* = 7). Other syndromes being mentioned by the included studies were Liver wind 肝风, Blood deficiency 血虚, *qi* deficiency 气虚 and cold stagnation 寒凝.

The names of CHM formulas were provided by 62 RCTs. In total 23 studies evaluated commercialised CHM products including pills, granules and capsules. The most common ones were *Zheng tian wan/ Zheng tian jiao nang* 正天丸/正天胶囊 (*n* = 5) and *Yang xue qing nao ke li* 养血清脑颗粒 (*n* = 4). The other 39 RCTs evaluated self-prescribed oral CHM formula decoctions; six studies did not provide a formula name. Of the formula names provided by the studies, only three formulas (of the same name) had been evaluated by multiple studies; these were *Chuan xiong cha tiao san* 川芎茶调散 (*n* = 3), modified *Jia Wei san pian tang*/*San pian tang ke li* 加味散偏汤/散偏汤颗粒 (*n* = 2) and *Chai shao zhi tong fang* 柴芍止痛方 (*n* = 2).

The pharmacotherapies for migraine prevention used in these studies as comparators were mainly of three categories: (1) calcium channel blockers (*n* = 50); (2) triptans (*n* = 1); and (3) antidepressants (*n* = 2). All these pharmacotherapies are recommended by clinical guidelines as the preventive treatments for migraine.[11]

The most frequently used herbs of all these oral CHM including products or decoctions were also analysed. See Table 5.1 for the most common formulas and Table 5.2 for the most common herbs.

Table 5.1. Frequently Reported Oral Formulas in Randomised Controlled Trials

Most Common Formulas	No. of Studies	Ingredients
Zheng tian wan/ Zheng tian jiao nang 正天丸/正天胶囊	5 (H7, H10, H41, H56, H59)	*Chuan xiong* 川芎, *dang gui* 当归, *bai shao* 白芍, *di huang* 地黄, *gou teng* 钩藤, *tao ren* 桃仁, *hong hua* 红花, *fu zi* 附子, *fang feng* 防风, *du huo* 独活, *ma huang* 麻黄, *ji xue teng* 鸡血藤 and *bai zhi* 白芷
Yang xue qing nao ke li 养血清脑颗粒	4 (H14, H27, H37, H38)	*Dang gui* 当归, *chuan xiong* 川芎, *bai shao* 白芍, *di huang* 地黄, *zhen zhu mu* 珍珠母 and *jue ming zi* 决明子
Chuan xiong cha tiao san 川芎茶调散	3 (H4, H48, H49)	*Chuan xiong* 川芎, *jing jie* 荆芥, *fang feng* 防风, *xi xin* 细辛, *qiang huo* 羌活, *bai zhi* 白芷, *bo he* 薄荷 and *gan cao* 甘草
San pian tang 散偏汤	2 (H26, H46)	*Chuan xiong* 川芎, *bai zhi* 白芷, *bai shao* 白芍, *bai jie zi* 白芥子, *xiang fu* 香附, *chai hu* 柴胡, *yu li ren* 郁李仁 and *gan cao* 甘草
Chai shao zhi tong fang 柴芍止痛方	2 (H39, H55)	*Chai hu* 柴胡, *bai shao* 白芍, *bai zhu* 白术, *dang gui* 当归, *chuang xiong* 川芎, *qing feng teng* 青风藤, *zhi ke* 枳壳 and *gan cao* 甘草

Ingredients are referenced to the *Zhong Yi Fang Ji Da Ci Dian* 中医方剂大辞典 where available, or to the included study if not available. The use of some herbs may be restricted in some countries. Readers are advised to comply with relevant regulations.

Table 5.2. Frequently Reported Orally Used Herbs in Randomised Controlled Trials for Migraine Prevention

Most Common Herbs	Scientific Name	Frequency of Use
Chuan xiong 川芎	*Ligusticum chuangxiong* Hort.	47
Bai zhi 白芷	*Angelica dahurica* (Fisch. ex Hoffm.) Benth. et Hook. f.	27
Bai shao 白芍	*Paeonia lactiflora* Pall.	26
Dang gui 当归	*Angelica sinensis* (Oliv.) Diels	22
Tian ma 天麻	*Gastrodia elata* Bl.	18
Xi xin 细辛	1. *Asarum heterotropoides* Fr. Schmidt var. *mandshuricum* (Maxim) Kitag. 2. *Asarum sieboldii* Miq. var. *seoulense* Nakai 3. *Asarum sieboldii* Miq.	18
Quan xie 全蝎	*Buthus martensii* Karsch	17
Tao ren 桃仁	1. *Prunus persica* (L.) Batsch 2. *Prunus davidiana* (Carr.) Franch	16
Gan cao 甘草	1. *Glycyrrhiza uralensis* Fisch. 2. *Glycyrrhiza inflata* Bat. 3. *Glycyrrhiza glabra* L.	15
Chai hu 柴胡	1. *Bupleurum chinense* DC. 2. *Bupleurum scorzonerifolium* Willd.	13
Gou teng 钩藤	*Uncaria rhynchophylla* (Miq.) Miq. ex Havil.	13
Hong hua 红花	*Carthamus tinctorius* L.	12
Man jing zi 蔓荆子	1. *Vitex trifolia* L. var. *simplicifolia* Cham. 2. *Vitex trifolia* L.	12
Di huang 地黄	*Rehmannia glutinosa Libosch.*	10
Fang feng 防风	*Saposhnikovia divaricata (Turcz.)* Schischk.	10
Shi jue ming 石决明	1. *Haliotis diversicolor* Reeve 2. *Haliotis discus hannai* Ino 3. *Haliotis ovina* Gmelin 4. *Haliotis ruber* (Leach) 5. *Haliotis asinina* L. 6. *Haliotis laevigata* (Donovan)	9

(Continued)

Table 5.2.   (*Continued*)

Most Common Herbs	Scientific Name	Frequency of Use
Qiang huo 羌活	*Notopterygium incisum* Ting ex H. T. Chang	9
Ge gen 葛根	*Pueraria lobata (Willd.) Ohwi*	9
Di long 地龙	1. *Pheretima aspergillum* (E. Perrier) 2. *Pheretima vulgaris* Chen 3. *Pheretima guillelmi* (Michaelsen) 4. *Pheretima pectinifera* Michaelsen	8
Dan shen 丹参	*Salvia miltiorrhiza* Bge.	7
Zhen zhu mu 珍珠母	1. *Hyriopsis cumingii* (Lea) 2. *Cristaria plicata* (Leach) 3. *Pteria martensii* (Dunker)	7

The use of some herbs may be restricted in some countries. Readers are advised to comply with relevant regulations.

Risk of Bias Assessment

Eighteen RCTs (H2, H3, H5, H6, H8, H9, H25, H33, H35, H36, H39, H44, H48, H51, H52, H55, H56, H60) applied appropriate randomisation sequence generation and therefore they were rated as 'low' risk of bias for sequence generation. Six studies (H11, H26, H41, H42, H45, H46) allocated participants based on their sequence of attending; they were assessed as 'high' risk of bias for this item. The remaining 38 studies were 'unclear' risk of bias for this since they did not provide sufficient information. For 'allocation conceal-ment', only two studies (H2, H25) were 'low' risk of bias, because they used opaque envelopes, the remaining 60 studies were 'unclear' risk of bias due to lack of information.

In terms of blinding (participants, personnel and outcome asses-sors), seven studies (H1, H2, H25, H32, H37, H41, H59) were assessed as 'low' risk of bias for these three items since they applied appropriate placebo control. Three studies (H7, H12, H60) were of 'unclear' risk of bias due to lack of information and the remaining studies were 'high' risk of bias because they compared CHM with other forms of therapies without design of placebo control.

In terms of incomplete outcome data, two studies (H6, H35) were judged as 'high' risk of bias because they had high drop-out rates and

Table 5.3. Risk of Bias of Randomised Controlled Trials: Oral Chinese Herbal Medicine for Migraine Prevention

Risk of Bias Domain	Low Risk n (%)	Unclear Risk n (%)	High Risk n (%)
Sequence generation	18(29.0)	38(61.3)	6(9.7)
Allocation concealment	2(3.2)	60(96.8)	0(0)
Blinding of participants	7(11.3)	3(4.8)	52(83.9)
Blinding of personnel	7(11.3)	3(4.8)	52(83.9)
Blinding of outcome assessors	7(11.3)	3(4.8)	52(83.9)
Incomplete outcome data	60(96.8)	0(0)	2(3.2)
Selective outcome reporting	0(0)	56(90.3)	6 (9.7)

did not use intention-to-treat (ITT) analysis to deal with missing data; the other 60 studies were of 'low' risk since their low drop-out rate or no drop-out did not affect the outcome results.

For selective reporting, six studies (H20, H23, H24, H27, H30, H57) were judged as 'high' risk of bias because they did not report all outcomes as stated in their methods section. The other 56 studies were 'unclear' risk of bias because they did not report publication or registration of their protocol. See Table 5.3 for details.

Outcomes

Outcome measures reported by these studies include migraine frequency (monthly), migraine days (monthly), migraine duration (monthly), pain visual analogue scale (VAS)/numeric rating scale (NRS), responder rate, acute medication usage and participants' quality of life (QoL). The treatment effects of CHM were analysed by pooling the studies of same comparison into meta-analyses. Details of results are shown below under each category of comparison:

- Oral CHM versus placebo (with, or without, pharmacotherapy as co-intervention in both groups) ($n = 10$);
- Oral CHM versus pharmacotherapy ($n = 37$);
- Oral CHM plus pharmacotherapy versus pharmacotherapy alone ($n = 15$).

Oral Chinese Herbal Medicine versus Placebo

Ten studies compared oral CHM with CHM placebo, with or without pharmacotherapy as co-intervention in both groups. Meta-analyses showed that, at the end of the treatment phase, the CHM group achieved greater effects than placebo for migraine frequency, migraine days, responder rate and pain VAS/NRS, but there was no significant difference between CHM and placebo for the duration of migraine and acute medication usage. At the end of the follow-up phase, CHM also showed superior effects than placebo for migraine duration, but not for migraine frequency (see Table 5.4).

Table 5.4. Oral Chinese Herbal Medicine versus Placebo

Outcome	No. of Studies	No. of Participants	Effect Size (MD or RR [95% CI], I^2)	Included Studies
Migraine frequency (monthly), end of treatment	5	453	MD: −2.05 [−3.75, −0.36]*, 99%	H2, H12, H32, H37, H41
Migraine frequency (monthly), end of follow-up	2	239	MD: −1.42 [−3.42, 0.59], 91%	H2, H32
Migraine days (monthly), end of treatment	4	287	MD: −1.43 [−2.22, −0.64]*, 74%	H2, H7, H25, H41
Responder rate, end of treatment	3	236	RR: 1.42 [1.04, 1.95]*, 65%	H1, H2, H59
Migraine duration, end of treatment	4	343	MD: −6.19 [−12.76, 0.38], 98%	H2, H12, H32, H41
Migraine duration, end of follow-up	2	239	MD: −11.34 [−18.66, −4.02]*, 0%	H2, H32
Pain VAS/NRS, end of treatment	3	224	MD: −0.99 [−1.39, −0.59]*, 0%	H2, H41, H60
Acute medication usage, end of treatment	2	184	MD: −0.07 [−0.27, 0.12], 0%	H2, H60

*Statistically significant.

Abbreviations: CI, confidence interval; MD, mean difference; NRS, numeric rating scale; RR, risk ratio; VAS, visual analogue scale.

Oral Chinese Herbal Medicine versus Pharmacotherapy

When comparing oral CHM with pharmacotherapy, it was found that at the end-of-treatment phase, oral CHM was more effective than pharmacotherapy for migraine frequency, migraine days, duration, responder rate, pain (VAS/NRS) and acute medication usage. At the end of the follow-up phase, oral CHM showed superior affects compared to pharmacotherapy for the outcomes of migraine frequency and acute medication usage, and there was no difference between oral CHM and pharmacotherapy for migraine days, duration and pain (VAS/NRS). Detailed results are presented in Table 5.5.

Table 5.5. Oral Chinese Herbal Medicine versus Pharmacotherapy

Outcome	No. of Studies	No. of Participants	Effect Size (MD or RR [95% CI], I^2)	Included Studies
Migraine frequency (monthly), end of treatment	21	1,591	MD: −1.58 [−2.13, −1.02]*, 98%	H3, H5, H8, H11, H13, H16, H20, H22–H24, H26, H35, H38, H42–H44, H46, H50, H56, H57, H62
Migraine frequency (monthly), end of follow-up	5	353	MD: −0.96 [−1.70, −0.21]*, 96%	H20, H42, H46, H56, H57
Migraine days (monthly), end of treatment	4	446	MD: −1.65 [−3.85, 0.54], 96%	H33, H46, H56, H57
Migraine days (monthly), end of follow-up	3	386	MD: −2.18 [−5.08, 0.72], 97%	H33, H46, H56
Responder rate, end of treatment	7	634	RR: 1.28 [1.15, 1.42]*, 36%	H14, H28, H33, H43, H56, H57, H61
Migraine duration, end of treatment	18	1381	MD: −1.99 [−3.13, −0.85]*, 92%	H5, H8, H11, H13, H15, H20, H22–H24, H26, H35, H36, H38, H42, H43, H50, H56, H62
Migraine duration, end of follow-up	4	322	MD: −2.80 [−6.11, 0.51], 97%	H20, H42, H50, H56

(Continued)

Table 5.5. (*Continued*)

Outcome	No. of Studies	No. of Participants	Effect Size (MD or RR [95% CI], I^2)	Included Studies
Pain VAS/NRS, end of treatment	14	1144	MD: −0.92 [−1.57, −0.26]*, 96%	H10, H13, H15, H18, H19, H21, H26, H35, H39, H43, H46–H48, H55
Pain VAS/NRS, end of follow-up	2	163	MD: −1.56 [−3.73, 0.61], 97%	H46, H56
Acute medication usage, end of treatment	5	506	MD: −0.70 [−1.24, −0.16]*, 95%	H3, H33, H42, H46, H56
Acute medication usage, end of follow-up	4	446	MD: −0.69 [−1.22, −0.15]*, 96%	H33, H42, H46, H56

*Statistically significant.
Abbreviations: CI, confidence interval; MD, mean difference; NRS, numeric rating scale; RR, risk ratio; VAS, visual analogue scale.

Oral Chinese Herbal Medicine plus Pharmacotherapy versus Pharmacotherapy Alone

When oral CHM was used as an add-on therapy in combination with pharmacotherapy and using the same pharmacotherapy as comparator, it was found by meta-analyses that adding oral CHM increased the effects for migraine frequency, migraine days, duration and pain (VAS/NRS). All these outcomes were assessed at the end-of-treatment phase. However, data of end of follow-up phase were lacking to prove the long-term benefits of adding CHM to pharmacotherapy. Detailed results are presented in Table 5.6.

Assessment Using Grading of Recommendations Assessment, Development and Evaluation

The certainty of evidence of overall oral CHM for migraine prevention are presented in Table 5.7 and Table 5.8. As shown in Table 5.7, when oral CHM was compared with placebo (with, or without,

Table 5.6. Oral Chinese Herbal Medicine plus Pharmacotherapy versus Pharmacotherapy Alone

Outcome	No. of Studies	No. of Participants	Effect Size (MD or RR [95% CI], I^2)	Included Studies
Migraine frequency (monthly), end of treatment	6	469	MD: −0.81 [−1.57, −0.05]*, 93%	H4, H9, H31, H34, H49, H51
Responder rate, end of treatment	4	369	RR: 1.43 [1.18, 1.72]*, 44%	H4, H17, H27, H51
Migraine duration, end of treatment	6	469	MD: −1.04 [−1.77, −0.32]*, 95%	H4, H9, H31, H34, H49, H51
Pain VAS/NRS, end of treatment	6	403	MD: −1.37 [−1.72, −1.03]*, 77%	H29, H31, H40, H45, H53, H54

*Statistically significant.

Abbreviations: CI, confidence interval; MD, mean difference; NRS, numeric rating scale; RR, risk ratio; VAS, visual analogue scale.

pharmacotherapy used as co-intervention in both groups) it was more effective than placebo for reducing the migraine frequency (monthly), migraine days (monthly) and pain, as well as improving responder rate. These were confirmed by meta-analysis of 'moderate' or 'low' certainty. When oral CHM was used as an add-on therapy, meta-analyses confirmed the effectiveness of adding CHM to reduce migraine frequency (monthly) and pain, as well as to improve responder rate. These evidences were assessed as of 'moderate' or 'low' certainty.

Randomised Controlled Trial Evidence for Individual Formulas

Four CHM formulas have been evaluated by multiple RCTs as the prevention treatment for migraine; these are *Zheng tian wan* or *Zheng tian jiao nang* 正天丸 (正天胶囊) (H7, H10, H41, H56, H59), *Yang xue qing nao ke li* 养血清脑颗粒 (H14, H27, H37, H38), *Chuan xiong cha tiao san* 川芎茶调散 (H4, H48, H49) and *Jia wei san pian tang* 加味散偏汤 (H26, H46). The treatment effects of these formulas

Table 5.7. GRADE: Oral Chinese Herbal Medicine (plus Pharmacotherapy) versus Placebo (plus Pharmacotherapy) for Migraine Prevention

Outcome	Estimated Absolute Effect		Relative Effect (95% CI) No. of Participants (Studies)	Certainty of the Evidence (GRADE)
	Oral CHM plus Pharmacotherapy	Placebo plus Pharmacotherapy		
Migraine frequency (monthly), end of treatment	**2.57** MD: 2.05 lower (95% CI: 3.75 lower to 0.36 lower)	**4.62**	**MD −2.05** (−3.75, −0.36) 453 (5 RCTs)	⊕⊕⊕◯ MODERATE[1]
Migraine frequency (monthly), end of follow-up	**1.63** MD: 1.42 lower (95% CI: 3.42 lower to 0.59 higher)	**3.05**	**MD −1.42** (−3.42, 0.59) 239 (2 RCTs)	⊕⊕◯◯ LOW[1,2]
Migraine days (monthly), end of treatment	**2.32** MD: 1.43 lower (95% CI: 2.22 to 0.64 lower)	**3.75**	**MD −1.43** (−2.22, −0.64) 287 (4 RCTs)	⊕⊕◯◯ LOW[1,2]
Migraine days (monthly), end of follow-up	**1.06** MD: 0.63 lower (95% CI: 1.6 lower to 0.34 higher)	**1.69**	**MD −0.63** (−1.6, +0.34) 128 (1 RCT)	⊕⊕⊕◯ MODERATE[2]
Responder rate, end of treatment	**84** per 100 Difference: 25 more per 100 patients (95% CI: 2 to 56 more per 100 patients)	**59** per 100	**RR 1.42** (1.04, 1.95) 236 (3 RCTs)	⊕⊕◯◯ LOW[1,2]

Pain VAS/NRS, end of treatment	**2.97** MD: 0.99 lower (95% CI: 1.39 to 0.59 lower)	3.96	**MD −0.99** (−1.39, −0.59) 224 (3 RCTs)	⊕⊕⊕◯ MODERATE[2]
Pain VAS/NRS, end of follow-up	**1.66** MD: 1.26 lower (95% CI: 2.14 to 0.38 lower)	2.92	**MD −1.26** (−2.14, −0.38) 128 (1 RCT)	⊕⊕⊕◯ MODERATE[2]

The risk in the intervention group (and its 95% confidence interval) is based on the assumed risk in the comparison group and the relative effect of the intervention (and its 95% CI).

Abbreviations: CHM, Chinese herbal medicine; CI, confidence interval; GRADE: Grading of Recommendations Assessment, Development and Evaluation; MD, mean difference; NRS, numeric rating scale; RCT(s), randomised controlled trial(s); RR, risk ratio; VAS, visual analogue scale/score.

Notes

[1]High heterogeneity may limit the certainty of results.
[2]Small sample size may limit the certainty of results.

Study references

Migraine frequency (monthly) (at the end of treatment): H2, H12, H32, H37, H41.
Migraine frequency (monthly) (at the end of follow-up): H2, H32.
Migraine days by month (at the end of treatment): H2, H7, H25, H41.
Migraine days by month (at the end of follow-up): H2.
Responder rate (at the end of treatment): H1, H2, H59.
Pain VAS/NRS (at the end of treatment): H2, H41, H60.
Pain VAS/NRS (at the end of follow-up): H2.

Table 5.8. GRADE: Oral Chinese Herbal Medicine plus Pharmacotherapy versus Pharmacotherapy Alone for Migraine Prevention

Outcome	Estimated Absolute Effect		Relative Effect (95% CI) No. of Participants (Studies)	Certainty of the Evidence (GRADE)
	Oral CHM plus Pharmacotherapy	Pharmacotherapy		
Migraine frequency (monthly), end of treatment	**2.01** MD: 0.81 lower (95% CI: 1.57 lower to 0.05 lower)	**2.82**	**MD −0.81** (−1.57, −0.05) 469 (6 RCTs)	⊕⊕○○ LOW[1,2]
Migraine days (monthly), end of treatment	**1.99** MD: 0.46 days lower (95% CI: 0.82 lower to 0.1 lower)	**2.45**	**MD −0.46** (−0.82, −0.1) 117 (1 RCT)	⊕⊕○○ LOW[1,3]
Responder rate, end of treatment	**79** per 100 Difference: 24 more per 100 patients (95% CI: 10 to 39 more per 100 patients)	**55** per 100	**RR 1.43** (1.18 to 1.72) 369 (4 RCTs)	⊕⊕⊕○ MODERATE[1]

Pain VAS/NRS, end of treatment	**2.53** MD: 1.37 lower (95% CI: 1.72 lower to 1.03 lower)	**3.9**	**MD −1.37** (−1.72, −1.03) 403 (6 RCTs)	⊕⊕○○ LOW[1,2]
MIDAS, end of treatment	**4.16** MD: 2.73 lower (95% CI: 3.24 lower to 2.22 lower)	**6.89**	**MD −2.73** (−3.24, −2.22) 121 (1 RCT)	⊕⊕○○ LOW[1,3]

The risk in the intervention group (and its 95% confidence interval) is based on the assumed risk in the comparison group and the relative effect of the intervention (and its 95% CI).

Abbreviations: CHM, Chinese herbal medicine; CI, confidence interval; GRADE: Grading of Recommendations Assessment, Development and Evaluation; MD, mean difference; MIDAS: Migraine Disability Assessment; NRS, numeric rating scale; RCT(s), randomised controlled trial(s); RR, risk ratio; VAS, visual analogue scale/score.

Notes

[1]High risk of bias in blinding may limit the certainty of the results.
[2]High heterogeneity may limit the certainty of the results.
[3]Small sample size may limit the certainty of results.

Study references

Migraine frequency (monthly) (at the end of treatment): H4, H9, H31, H34, H49, H51.
Migraine days by month (at the end of treatment): H4.
Responder rate (at the end of treatment): H4, H17, H27, H51.
Pain VAS/NRS (at the end of treatment): H29, H31, H40, H45, H53, H54.
MIDAS (at the end of treatment): H30.

were analysed and results of meta-analyses are presented here. The data of studies evaluating *Yang xue qing nao ke li* 养血清脑颗粒 could not be pooled for meta-analysis due to the diversity of comparison and outcomes.

Zheng Tian Wan or Zheng Tian Jiao Nang 正天丸 (正天胶囊)

Zheng tian wan 正天丸 and *Zheng tian jiao nang* 正天胶囊 are commercialised CHM products which were formulated for reducing headaches including migraine. The main ingredients are *gou teng* 钩藤, *bai shao* 白芍, *chuan xiong* 川芎, *dang gui* 当归, *di huang* 地黄, *bai zhi* 白芷, *fang feng* 防风, *qiang huo* 羌活, *tao ren* 桃仁, *hong hua* 红花, *xi xin* 细辛, *du huo* 独活, *ma huang* 麻黄, *fu zi* 附子 and *ji xue teng* 鸡血藤.

When *Zheng tian wan* or *Zheng tian jiao nang* 正天丸 (正天胶囊) is compared with placebo CHM, the CHM was more effective for the number of migraine days at the end of treatment phase (two studies, MD: −1.42 [−2.41, −0.43], I^2 = 70%) (H7, H41). The certainty of this evidence was assessed as 'low' using Grading of Recommendations Assessment, Development and Evaluation (GRADE) assessment. When *Zheng tian wan* or *Zheng tian jiao nang* 正天丸 (正天胶囊) was compared with pharmacotherapy, it was also more effective for reducing migraine days at the end-of-treatment phase (two studies, MD: −0.64 [−1.08, −0.20], I^2 = 0%) (H10, H56), with the certainty of this evidence being assessed as 'low' using GRADE assessment. For other outcomes, there was not poolable data for meta-analysis.

Chuan Xiong Cha Tiao San 川芎茶调散

Meta-analyses of two studies (H4, H49) showed that adding *Chuan xiong cha tiao san* 川芎茶调散 to pharmacotherapy did not achieve superior effects than pharmacotherapy alone at the end-of-treatment phase for the outcome of migraine frequency (MD: −0.01 [−1.53, 1.51], I^2 = 96%).

The certainty of evidence for this outcome was assessed as 'very low' by GRADE assessment.

Jia Wei San Pian Tang 加味散偏汤

Outcome data of pain VAS and migraine frequency at the end-of-treatment phase were reported by the two studies (H26, H46) that compared *Jia wei san pian tang* 加味散偏汤 to pharmacotherapy. It was found that the CHM *Jia wei san pian tang* 加味散偏汤 was more effective than pharmacotherapy (VAS; MD: −1.88 [−3.14, −0.62], I^2 = 92%; migraine frequency; MD: −1.72 [−2.44, −0.99], I^2 = 89%). Both these two meta-analyses were assessed as 'very low' certainty by the GRADE assessment.

Frequently Reported Herbs in Meta-analyses Showing Favourable Effect

In order to show which herbs contributed to the meta-analyses with favourable effects towards oral CHM, the studies included in those meta-analyses were pooled for herb frequency analyses. Since there were multiple meta-analyses of different comparisons and different outcomes, these herb analyses were based on outcomes in the same category regardless of the comparisons and the time point of outcome assessment. Outcomes are grouped as four main categories:

- Migraine frequency, migraine duration and migraine days: all these are calculated on a monthly base;
- Responder rate;
- Migraine pain VAS/NRS;
- Acute medication usage.

Results are shown in the Table 5.9.

There were 37 RCTs included in six meta-analyses which achieved significant favourable effects of migraine frequency and duration days. The most frequently used herbs in studies included were *chuan xiong* 川芎, *bai zhi* 白芷, *bai shao* 白芍, *tao ren* 桃仁, *xi xin* 细辛, *quan xie* 全蝎, *tian ma* 天麻, *dang gui* 当归, *gan cao* 甘草 and *gou teng* 钩藤.

Table 5.9.   Frequently Reported Orally Used Herbs in Meta-analyses Showing Favourable Effect for Migraine Prevention

Outcome Measure	No. of Meta-analyses	No. of Studies	Herbs	Scientific Name	Frequency of Use
Migraine frequency, migraine duration, migraine days (monthly)	6	37	Chuan xiong 川芎	Ligusticum chuangxiong Hort.	28
			Bai zhi 白芷	Angelica dahurica (Fisch. ex Hoffm.) Benth. et Hook. f.	17
			Bai shao 白芍	Paeonia lactiflora Pall.	14
			Tao ren 桃仁	1. Prunus persica (L.) Batsch 2. Prunus davidiana (Carr.) Franch	11
			Xi xin 细辛	1. Asarum heterotropoides Fr. Schmidt var. mandshuricum (Maxim) Kitag. 2. Asarum sieboldii Miq. var. seoulense Nakai 3. Asarum sieboldii Miq.	11
			Quan xie 全蝎	Buthus martensii Karsch	10
			Tian ma 天麻	Gastrodia elata Bl.	10
			Dang gui 当归	Angelica sinensis (Oliv.) Diels	9
			Gan cao 甘草	1. Glycyrrhiza uralensis Fisch. 2. Glycyrrhiza inflata Bat. 3. Glycyrrhiza glabra L.	8
			Gou teng 钩藤	Uncaria rhynchophylla (Miq.) Miq. ex Havil.	8
Responder rate	1	14	Chuan xiong 川芎	Ligusticum chuangxiong Hort.	10
			Dang gui 当归	Angelica sinensis (Oliv.) Diels	5
			Bai shao 白芍	Paeonia lactiflora Pall.	5

			Xi xin 细辛	1. *Asarum heterotropoides* Fr. Schmidt var. *mandshuricum* (Maxim) Kitag. 2. *Asarum sieboldii* Miq. var. *seoulense* Nakai 3. *Asarum sieboldii* Miq.	5
			Di huang 地黄	*Rehmannia glutinosa Libosch.*	4
			Bai zhi 白芷	*Angelica dahurica* (Fisch. ex Hoffm.) Benth. et Hook. f.	4
			Quan xie 全蝎	*Buthus martensii Karsch*	3
			Tao ren 桃仁	1. *Prunus persica* (L.) Batsch 2. *Prunus davidiana* (Carr.) Franch	3
			Hong hua 红花	*Carthamus tinctorius L.*	3
			Qiang huo 羌活	*Notopterygium incisum* Ting ex H. T. Chang	3
			Gou teng 钩藤	*Uncaria rhynchophylla* (Miq.) Miq. ex Havil.	3
			Fang feng 防凤	*Saposhnikovia divaricata (Turcz.) Schischk.*	3
Migraine pain intensity, VAS/NRS	2	24	Chuan xiong 川芎	*Ligusticum chuangxiong Hort.*	17
			Bai zhi 白芷	*Angelica dahurica* (Fisch. ex Hoffm.) Benth. et Hook. f.	13
			Bai shao 白芍	*Paeonia lactiflora Pall.*	12
			Dang gui 当归	*Angelica sinensis (Oliv.) Diels*	11
			Chai hu 柴胡	1. *Bupleurum chinense* DC. 2. *Bupleurum scorzonerifolium* Willd.	7

(Continued)

Table 5.9. (*Continued*)

Outcome Measure	No. of Meta-analyses	No. of Studies	Herbs	Scientific Name	Frequency of Use
			Tian ma 天麻	Gastrodia elata Bl.	6
			Xi xin 细辛	1. Asarum heterotropoides Fr. Schmidt var. mandshuricum (Maxim) Kitag. 2. Asarum sieboldii Miq. var. seoulense Nakai 3. Asarum sieboldii Miq.	6
			Gou teng 钩藤	Uncaria rhynchophylla (Miq.) Miq. ex Havil.	6
			Fang feng 防风	Saposhnikovia divaricata (Turcz.) Schischk.	6
			Gan cao 甘草	1. Glycyrrhiza uralensis Fisch. 2. Glycyrrhiza inflata Bat. 3. Glycyrrhiza glabra L.	5
Acute medication usage	2	5	Chuan xiong 川芎	Ligusticum chuangxiong Hort.	4
			Chai hu 柴胡	Bupleurum chinense DC.	3
			Gan cao 甘草	1. Glycyrrhiza uralensis Fisch. 2. Glycyrrhiza inflata Bat. 3. Glycyrrhiza glabra L.	3
			Bai zhi 白芷	Angelica dahurica (Fisch. ex Hoffm.) Benth. et Hook. f.	3

The use of some herbs may be restricted in some countries. Readers are advised to comply with relevant regulations.

Abbreviations: NRS, numeric rating scale; VAS, visual analogue scale.

In terms of responder rate, 14 RCTs were included in one meta-analysis showing favourable effects of oral CHM. The most frequent herbs used by these studies were *chuan xiong* 川芎, *dang gui* 当归, *bai shao* 白芍, *xi xin* 细辛, *di huang* 地黄, *bai zhi* 白芷, *quan xie* 全蝎, *tao ren* 桃仁, *hong hua* 红花, *qiang huo* 羌活, *gou teng* 钩藤 and *fang feng* 防风.

When pooling the studies which contributed to the positive meta-analysis of pain VAS/NRS, the most frequently used herbs were *chuan xiong* 川芎, *bai zhi* 白芷, *bai shao* 白芍, *dang gui* 当归, *chai hu* 柴胡, *tian ma* 天麻, *xi xin* 细辛, *gou teng* 钩藤 *fang feng* 防风 and *gan cao* 甘草.

At the end, the studies included in the meta-analyses showing favourable effects of CHM for reducing acute medication usage were pooled. Frequently used herbs in these studies were *chuan xiong* 川芎, *chai hu* 柴胡, *gan cao* 甘草 and *bai zhi* 白芷. In fact, all these herbs are also included in the most frequent herbs of all included RCTs (see Table 5.2) and there is no significant diversity across different pools based on outcome categories. This could be explained by the fact that the CHM formulas were not designed to be effective for any specific outcome measure; using oral CHM would generally benefit migraine sufferers.

Controlled Clinical Trials (Non-randomised) of Oral Chinese Herbal Medicine

Two non-randomised CCTs were identified from our search (H64, H65). Both studies compared oral CHM to flunarizine capsule as preventive treatment of migraine. One study (H64) evaluated the oral CHM product *Zheng tian wan* 正天丸 and the other study (H65) used CHM decoction *Huo xue zhi tong tang* 活血止痛汤. A total of 174 participants were involved. Treatment duration was eight weeks (H65) and four weeks (H64). Both studies reported pain VAS at the end-of-treatment phase. Meta-analysis showed that there was no significant difference between oral CHM and flunarizine for pain VAS (MD: 0.08 [−2.39, 2.55], I^2 = 98%). Safety information was not reported in these studies.

Non-controlled Clinical Studies of Oral Chinese Herbal Medicine

Three non-controlled clinical studies (H66, H67, H68) were identified from our search; two studies were case series studies (H66, H67) involving 169 patients and the other study (H68) was a case report. More female than male patients were involved (110 versus 60). Oral CHM *Yang xue qing nao ke li* 养血清脑颗粒 (H66), *Chuan xiong qing nao ke li* 川芎清脑颗粒 (H67) and *Xie xin tang* 泻心汤 (H68) were reported effective for the prevention and management for migraine. Safety information of oral CHM was not reported by these studies.

Oral Chinese Herbal Medicine for Acute Migraine Management

Two RCTs (H30, H63) compared the combination of oral CHM and pharmacotherapy to pharmacotherapy alone for acute migraine management. One study (H30) used oral CHM *Tong luo qing kong tang* 通络清空汤 for both prevention and acute management for migraine and the other study (H63) only evaluated the effects of oral *Yang xue qing nao ke li* 养血清脑颗粒 for acute migraine management. A total of 223 participants were involved in these studies. Outcome data reported by these two studies were for responder rate, pain VAS/NRS and Migraine Disability Assessment (MIDAS) score. However, the treatment effects could not be confirmed by meta-analysis since there were no poolable data.

Safety of Oral Chinese Herbal Medicine

Of all included RCTs, 42 studies reported information of AEs. Among them, 17 studies (H3–H6, H12, H14, H16–H18, H39, H41, H42, H52, H57–H60) reported that there were no AEs observed during the entire trial and 25 studies (H1, H2, H10, H15, H21–H26, H31, H32, H35–H37, H40, H43, H46, H48, H50, H51, H53, H55, H56, H61) reported mild or moderate AEs being observed. Overall there were more AEs reported in the control groups than those of the CHM groups (102 cases versus 71 cases). The AEs reported by the CHM treatment groups were mild gastrointestinal symptoms; usually these symptoms ceased by adjusting the time and dosage of medicine and no additional medical attention was required. There were two cases of severe AEs reported by the control group (H37, H48); one required additional medical care (H48) and the other one dropped out the trial because of the AE (H37). The other AEs reported by the control group were all mild or moderate.

In the studies that evaluated the add-on effects of CHM, the AEs of the CHM plus pharmacological therapy group were less than those reported by the pharmacological therapy alone group. Authors of these studies commonly stated that adding CHM to pharmacological therapy could reduce the AEs caused by the pharmacological therapy. In the studies that compared CHM with pharmacological therapy, it seems that the AEs caused by CHM were less than those caused by pharmacological therapy. In addition to the RCTs, information of AEs was reported in one CCT (H65), that there were only mild gastrointestinal symptoms observed in both treatment and control groups, without any medical treatment needed.

Evidence for Oral Chinese Herbal Medicine Treatments Commonly Used in Clinical Practice

The common practice of CHM treatment for migraine recommended by clinical guidelines and textbooks is summarised in Chapter 2. Many of the CHM formulas presented in Chapter 2 have not been evaluated by clinical studies. For example, the oral CHM formulas *Tian ma gou teng yin* 天麻钩藤饮, *Ban xia bai zhu tian ma tang* 半夏白术天麻汤, *Ba zhen tang* 八珍汤, *Qi ju di huang wan* 杞菊地黄丸 and *Wu zhu yu tang* 吴茱萸汤, and the commercialised CHM products *Tong tian kou fu ye* 通天口服液, *Fu fang yang jiao pian* 复方羊角片 or *Fu fang yang jiao ke li* 复方羊角颗粒, *Xue fu zhu yu kou fu ye* 血府逐瘀口服液, *Xue fu zhu yu jiao nang* 血府逐瘀胶囊 and *Tian ma tou tong pian* 天麻头痛片 have not been evaluated by any clinical studies included in our evaluation. The formulas listed below are the oral CHM formulas or products which were recommended in Chapter 2 and also have obtained evidence from clinical studies:

Zheng Tian Wan 正天丸 *and Yang Xue Qing Nao Ke Li* 养血清脑颗粒

These two products have been evaluated by multiple RCTs for migraine prevention; see above for details. In addition, there was one CCT (H64) that evaluated the treatment effects of *Zheng tian wan* 正天丸 to prevent migraine, one CCT (H63) that evaluated the effects of *Yang xue qing nao ke li* 养血清脑颗粒 for acute migraine and one non-controlled study (H66) that reported the effects of *Yang xue qing nao ke li* 养血清脑颗粒 for migraine prevention.

Tong Qiao Huo Xue Tang 通窍活血汤

One RCT (H5) that included 117 participants compared *Tong qiao huo xue tang* 通窍活血汤 to flunarizine for a four-week treatment phase and reported data on migraine frequency and duration at the end of treatment.

Quan Tian Ma Jiao Nang 全天麻胶囊

The CHM product *Quan tian ma jiao nang* 全天麻胶囊 was not evaluated by any included study. A product named *Tian ma su* 天麻素 containing gastrodin, which was extracted from the CM herb *tian ma* 天麻, was used in one RCT (H15) with 84 participants being involved to evaluate its add-on effects to flunarizine. Pain VAS and migraine duration were reported as outcome measures. Except for oral CHM, there are other forms of CHM therapies also recommended in Chapter 2, including CHM sniffing, CHM external application and CHM fumigation and steaming therapy. There is no evidence from clinical studies included in our evaluation to support the use of these therapies.

Summary of Oral Chinese Herbal Medicine Clinical Evidence

The evaluation of the clinical study evidence found variation in formulas of CHM and diversity in outcomes reported. Oral CHM was the most frequently investigated form of administration and the only form included in our evaluation.

Based on our evaluation, previously published systematic reviews suggested that oral CHM *Chuan xiong cha tiao san* 川芎茶调散, *Yang xue qing nao ke li* 养血清脑颗粒, *Xue fu zhu yu tang* 血府逐淤汤, *Tong xin luo jiao nang* 通心络胶囊, *Tou tong ning* 头痛宁, *Du liang ruan jiao nang* 都梁软胶囊 and other unnamed CHM formulas were effective for preventing migraine, for a group of outcome measures.

Most of the clinical studies included in our evaluation investigated oral CHM for preventing migraine; only two studies investigated the effects of oral CHM for acute migraine attack. For preventing migraine, there were almost 30 oral CHM decoction formulas and 16 commercialised oral CHM products being assessed. *Zheng tian wan/ Zheng tian jiao nang* 正天丸/正天胶囊 and *Yang xue qing nao ke li* 养血清脑颗粒 were the most frequently evaluated CHM treatments, with *Zheng tian wan/Zheng tian jiao nang* 正天丸/正天胶囊 only used for migraine prevention and *Yang xue qing nao ke li* 养血清脑颗粒 used for both prevention and acute migraine management. Chinese medicine syndrome information was reported by less than half of the included studies, with Blood stasis 瘀血阻滞 and Liver *yang* uprising 肝阳上亢 being the most commonly reported syndromes. The average treatment duration of using CHM was around 50 days for migraine prevention, but it is unclear for treating acute migraine due to lack of evidence.

In terms of the most frequently used herbs in the oral CHM treatment for migraine prevention, it was found that the herbs used in all RCTs (Table 5.2) are consistent with those shown in the studies of meta-analyses showing favourable effects (Table 5.9). Furthermore, the frequent herbs of RCTs included in meta-analyses showing favourable effects in terms of different outcomes are also consistent;

it was not distinguishable what herbs were effective for a particular outcome (Table 5.7).

In terms of the most frequently used herbs (see the most frequently used herbs in Table 5.2), it was found that the most common functions of these herbs were (1) eliminating wind (e.g. *chuan xiong* 川芎, *bai zhi* 白芷, *tian ma* 天麻, *xi xin* 细辛, *gou teng* 钩藤, *fang feng* 防风, *shi jue ming* 石决明, *qiang huo* 羌活 and *di long* 地龙); (2) activating and nourishing Blood and removing Blood stasis (e.g. *chuan xiong* 川芎, *dang gui* 当归, *tao ren* 桃仁, *hong hua* 红花, *bai shao* 白芍 and *di huang* 地黄); (3) reducing pain (e.g. *chuan xiong* 川芎, *bai zhi* 白芷, *bai shao* 白芍, *dang gui* 当归, *xi xin* 细辛, *quan xie* 全蝎, *man jing zi* 蔓荆子, *qiang huo* 羌活, *ge gen* 葛根 and *dan shen* 丹参); and (4) calming Liver and suppressing *yang* (e.g. *bai shao* 白芍, *tian ma* 天麻, *gou teng* 钩藤, *shi jue ming* 石决明 and *zhen zhu mu* 珍珠母). The use of these herbs reflected the common CM syndromes and corresponding treatment principles of migraine, that is, wind attack, Blood stasis 瘀血阻滞 and Liver *yang* uprising 肝阳上亢.

In terms of treatment effects, promising clinical evidence was seen with oral CHM formulas and products for migraine prevention. It was shown by meta-analyses that:

- Oral CHM was more effective than placebo for migraine frequency, migraine days, responder rate and pain VAS/NRS at the end-of-treatment phase;
- Oral CHM was more effective than clinical guideline-recommended pharmacotherapy for migraine frequency, migraine days, migraine duration, responder rate, pain VAS/NRS and acute medication usage at the end-of-treatment phase;
- Oral CHM was more effective than clinical guideline-recommended pharmacotherapy for migraine frequency and acute medication usage at the end of follow-up phase;
- Oral CHM was more effective when it was used as an add-on therapy to pharmacotherapy for migraine frequency, migraine days, migraine duration and pain VAS/NRS at the end-of-treatment phase.

The effects of oral CHM for migraine patients' QoL were not supported by our evaluation, since data on QoL outcomes were seldom reported.

Our evaluation found that there was meta-analyses evidence showing superior effects of *Zheng tian wan* or *Zheng tian jiao nang* 正天丸/正天胶囊 and *Jia wei san pian tang* 加味散偏汤 to pharmacotherapy; however, adding *Chuan xiong cha tiao san* 川芎茶调散 to pharmacotherapy did not achieve superior effects compared to pharmacotherapy alone. Nevertheless, the number of studies included in these meta-analyses were very small and therefore these results could not be confirmed. Meta-analysis evidence to support the use of *Yang xue qing nao ke li* 养血清脑颗粒 is lacking.

Using the GRADE approach, all the abovementioned meta-analyses results were assessed as 'low' to 'moderate' certainty. The common reasons for downgrading the certainty were high risk of bias in blinding, high heterogeneity and/small sample size. On the other hand, oral CHM was proved to be safe to be used as migraine management. However, there was insufficient evidence supporting the use of CHM for acute migraine. In addition, our evaluation did not find any evidence supporting the use of other forms of administration of CHM for the management of migraine.

In summary, there is promising evidence supporting the use of oral CHM for preventing migraine, in terms of reducing the monthly migraine frequency and days, the duration and pain of migraine attacks and the use of acute medication usage. Long-term effects of oral CHM were also seen for reducing migraine frequency and acute medication usage.

References

1. 史琳. (2011) 中医药治疗偏头痛的meta-分析 (Thesis). 山东中医药大学.
2. 谢炜. (2011) 中药与西药对照治疗偏头痛的 meta 分析. 热带医学杂志 **11(3):** 264–267.
3. Higgins J, Green S. (2011) Cochrane handbook for systematic reviews of interventions version 5.1.0. The Cochrane collaboration. Confidence intervals.

4. 曾敬. (2013) 通心络胶囊治疗偏头痛的系统评价. 西部中医药 **26(4):** 62–65.

5. 谭华威. (2014) 头痛宁治疗偏头痛效果及安全性的 meta 分析. 中国医药导报 **11(30):** 65–69.

6. 陈欢. (2014) 头痛宁与西药治疗偏头痛有效性与安全性的 meta 分析. 中国现代医药杂志 **16(12):** 1–4.

7. Xiao Y, Yuan L, Liu Y, *et al.* (2015) Traditional Chinese patent medicine for prophylactic treatment of migraine: A meta-analysis of randomized, double-blind, placebo-controlled trials. *Eur J Neurol* **22(2):** 361–368.

8. 王凤姣. (2016) 都梁软胶囊治疗瘀阻脑络型无先兆偏头痛的临床研究 (Thesis). 北京中医药大学.

9. 赖星. (2017) 中医药对比氟桂利嗪治疗偏头痛的疗效评价和 meta 分析 (Thesis). 湖北中医药大学.

10. 闫杨杨. (2017) 中药与西药对照治疗肝阳上亢型偏头痛的 meta 分析. 云南中医中药杂志 **38(4):** 14–17.

11. 中国偏头痛防治指南. (2016) 中国疼痛医学杂志 **22(10):** 721–727.

References to Included Studies

H1 陈鸿雁. (2015) 平肝潜阳, 活血化瘀法治疗无先兆偏头痛缓解期 (肝阳上亢挟血瘀型) 的临床研究 (Thesis). 长春中医药大学.

H2 付彩红. (2013) 川芎定痛饮治疗偏头痛肝风挟瘀证的疗效特点研究. 北京中医药大学 **23(15):** 255–256.

H3 马洁德. (2014) 柴胡桂枝干姜汤加减治疗偏头痛 (肝郁脾虚证) 的临床疗效观察 (Thesis). 山东中医药大学.

H4 聂长勇, 何昌生. (2015) 中西医结合治疗偏头痛 (风寒兼瘀证) 临床观察. 中国中医急症 **24(8):** 1435–1437.

H5 钱玉良, 严冬. (2006) 通窍活血汤治疗偏头痛 57 例临床观察. 湖南中医杂志 **22(6):** 6–8.

H6 僧志飞. (2015) 消痛方治疗偏头痛 (寒凝血瘀型) 的临床研究: 河南中医学院.

H7 王爽. (2008) 正天丸治疗偏头痛 (血虚阳亢挟瘀证) 的临床研究. 长春中医药大学.

H8 王琰. (2013) 平肝祛风通络法治疗肝阳上亢型偏头痛 58 例. 河南中医 **33(6):** 921–922.

H9 王琰. (2013) 中西医结合治疗偏头痛 42 例临床观察. 中医药导报 **19(3):** 106–107.

(*Continued*)

H10	张萍. (2013) 正天丸治疗瘀血阻络型偏头痛的临床研究 (Thesis). 南京中医药大学.
H11	钟广伟, 李炜, 罗艳红, *et al.* (2009) 平肝潜阳药物对偏头痛肝阳上亢证患者的临床疗效及其对血淋巴细胞蛋白质表达的影响. 中西医结合学报 **7(01):** 25–33.
H12	周永红, 张雅萍, 王新陆. (2003) 开郁宁脑胶囊治疗偏头痛临床研究. 安徽中医临床杂志 **15(3):** 189–190.
H13	富高研. (2015) 祛风活血方防治偏头痛的临床研究. 中医临床研究 **7(11):** 101–102.
H14	王梅. (2007) 养血清脑颗粒治疗偏头痛的临床观察. 中国医院用药评价与分析 **7(3):** 228–229.
H15	朱尤来. (2006) 基层医学论坛 **10(4):** 312–313.
H16	蔡之幸, 陈越, 王重卿, *et al.* (2017) 理虚祛风通络方治疗无先兆偏头痛. 吉林中医药 **37(12):** 1237–1239.
H17	陈伏建, 黄健飞, 方欣荣, 于晓月. (2013) 麝香保心丸开窍化瘀功能在治疗偏头痛中的增效作用观察. 浙江中医药大学学报 **37(2):** 166–168.
H18	陈杰. (2010) 以西比灵对照评价芎芷镇痛方治疗偏头痛的临床疗效 (Thesis). 南京中医药大学.
H19	陈戎. (2011) 天麻活血通络汤治疗偏头痛 90 例临床研究. 山东中医杂志 **30(8):** 544–545.
H20	代彪晖. (2005) 血塞通软胶囊治疗偏头痛 36 例疗效观察. 中国中医药信息杂志 **12(4):** 65–66.
H21	杜青. (2014) 芎芷煎方治疗偏头痛肝风挟瘀证的疗效评价及作用机理研究 (Thesis). 南京中医药大学.
H22	杜彦侠, 杨立波, 马静, 杨超. (2011) 从络病论治偏头痛的临床观察. 中华中医药杂志 **26(7):** 1652–1653.
H23	高焕民, 柳耀泉, 王少萍. (2006) 天舒胶囊治疗偏头痛 40 例. 中成药 **28(5):** 680–682.
H24	高建苑, 孙静, 吴利平, 孟华. (2009) 中药治疗女性偏头痛临床观察. 中國中醫急症 **18(04):** 507+531.
H25	葛鑫宇. (2009) 川芎油软胶囊治疗偏头痛的临床观察及疗效分析 (Thesis). 南方医科大学.
H26	苟成钢, 苗治国. (2014) 散偏汤预防性治疗偏头痛寒凝血瘀证的疗效观察. 中国实用神经疾病杂志 **17(16):** 52–53.
H27	何平, 陈晓玲. (2002) 养血清脑颗粒联合氟桂利嗪治疗偏头痛的临床观察. 中国临床康复 **16:** 2462.

(*Continued*)

(Continued)

H28   黄宏强, 杨荣源, 赵亚星. (2006) 通络法治疗偏头痛 30 例疗效观察. 新中医 **38(10):** 46–47.

H29   黄玉龙, 丁培杰, 马福云, 李枝锦. (2016) 麻黄附子细辛汤联合盐酸氟桂利嗪胶囊治疗偏头痛疗效观察. 中国中医急症 **25(9):** 1816–1818.

H30   吉贞料, 卢桂兰, 王高岸. (2016) 通络清空汤辨治偏头痛急性发作期的疗效及作用机制. 中国实验方剂学杂志 **22(19):** 154–158.

H31   李伯英, 何海洲. (2012) 养阴化湿活血汤联合阿米替林治疗偏头痛疗效观察. 现代中西医结合杂志 **21(30):** 3381–3382.

H32   李大年, 崔元孝. (1994) 中药静痛灵胶囊防治偏头痛的双盲安慰剂对照研究. 临床神经病学杂志 **7(4):** 197–199.

H33   梁斌. (2015) 和解止痛方治疗偏头痛肝郁脾虚证的临床研究 (Thesis). 长春中医药大学.

H34   梁建. (2013) 平肝通络法治疗偏头痛临床观察. 内蒙古中医药 **32(34):** 29.

H35   刘婷婷. (2009) 头痛安方治疗偏头痛痰热上扰证的临床研究 (Thesis). 新疆医科大学.

H36   罗俊超, 舒劲松. (2013) 自拟头痛汤治疗偏头痛 32 例疗效观察. 国际中医中药杂志 **35(3):** 248–249.

H37   罗盛, 王新德, 匡培根, *et al.* (2001) 养血清脑颗粒预防和治疗偏头痛的临床研究. 中华神经科杂志 **34(5):** 291–294.

H38   牛争平, 侯玉立, 任旭. (2003) 养血清脑颗粒对偏头痛病人头痛发作的影响研究. 中西医结合心脑血管病杂志 **1(6):** 327–329.

H39   毛丽军, 吴平凡, 刘红梅. (2011) 解郁祛风通络法治疗偏头痛临床观察. 中西医结合心脑血管病杂志 **9(06):** 693–694.

H40   马娟, 刘宁, 陈军, *et al.* (2013) 头痛宁胶囊联合氟桂利嗪胶囊治疗偏头痛的临床疗效及机理研究. 中成药 **35(04):** 677–680.

H41   梅群丽. (2010) 正天丸对偏头痛 (风瘀候) 的临床研究 (Thesis). 湖北中医药大学.

H42   潘平康, 陈亮, 马岱朝, *et al.* (2015) 加减芎龙汤分经论治对偏头痛预防性治疗的临床研究. 陕西中医 **36(11):** 1464–1466.

H43   彭祖春. (2017) 偏头痛患者采用中医内科治疗的效果观察. 中西医结合心血管病电子杂志 **5(01):** 1–2.

H44   曲淼, 唐启盛, 裴清华, 李侠. (2010) 温阳降气法治疗偏头痛的随机对照临床研究. 世界中联第三届中医中西医结合老年医学学术大会. 中国河南南阳.

H45   商建飞, 许旭东. (2016) 元胡止痛胶囊辅助治疗偏头痛临床观察. 医药前沿 **6(14):** 330–331.

(*Continued*)

H46 申斌, 于川, 王磊, *et al.* (2016) 加味散偏汤颗粒剂治疗偏头痛肝郁血瘀型 60 例. 中国中医药现代远程教育 **14(04):** 51–54.

H47 宋述强. (2017) 中医辨证治疗偏头痛32例. 广西中医药 **40(05):** 12–13.

H48 孙达, 许保海. (2016) 川芎茶调散治疗偏头痛的疗效观察及对 β 内啡肽、五羟色胺的影响. 中国中医急症 **25(11):** 2117–2119.

H49 孙宏建, 郭燕洁, 孙小涵. (2015) 中西医结合治疗偏头痛 30 例. 河南中医 **35(11):** 2828–2830.

H50 王改凤, 李文涛, 王松龄. (2012) 散寒活瘀止痛方治疗阳虚寒凝型偏头痛 60 例疗效观察. 新中医 **44(12):** 22–23.

H51 王国栋. (2011) 松龄血脉康联合氟桂利嗪治疗偏头痛疗效观察. 中华全科医师杂志 **10(7):** 525–526.

H52 王铃清. (2016) 自拟柔肝熄风汤对肝阳上亢型偏头痛预防性治疗疗效的临床研究 (Thesis). 河南中医药大学.

H53 王琼琼, 巩固. (2017) 中西医结合治疗偏头痛的效果研究. 中医临床研究 **9(13):** 85–86.

H54 翁旭亮. (2015) 止痛平风汤联合氟桂利嗪治疗偏头痛33例临床观察. 中国民族民间医药 **24(12):** 79–80.

H55 吴平凡. (2009) 解郁祛风通络法治疗偏头痛的临床研究 (Thesis). 北京中医药大学.

H56 谢颖兰. (2015) 正天胶囊治疗偏头痛风阳挟瘀型的临床研究 (Thesis). 湖北中医药大学.

H57 辛林娜. (2016) 头痛方治疗偏头痛 (气虚血瘀型) 的临床研究 (Thesis). 长春中医药大学.

H58 袁爱芹. (2017) 清热燥湿和解少阳法在偏头痛临床治疗中的疗效观察 (Thesis). 山东中医药大学.

H59 原志秋. (2014) 正天胶囊治疗偏头痛血虚阳亢挟瘀证的临床研究 (Thesis). 长春中医药大学.

H60 翟盼. (2016) 息风止痛颗粒治疗偏头痛血虚风动证的临床研究 (Thesis). 湖北中医药大学.

H61 翟穗燕, 陈锐, 吴学红. (2006) 复方丹参滴丸治疗偏头痛 41 例观察. 实用中医药杂志 **22(01):** 26.

H62 张轶丹. (2014) 平肝潜阳、化瘀通络法治疗肝阳上亢型偏头痛的疗效观察. 中国医药指南 **12(18):** 281–282.

H63 赵军. (2013) 养血清脑颗粒联合氟桂利嗪治疗急性发作期偏头痛 55 例. 陕西中医 **34(11):** 1475–1476.

(*Continued*)

(*Continued*)

H64 梁天山, 吴艳华, 徐念. (2015) 正天丸治疗瘀血阻络型偏头痛临床疗效观察. 中医临床研究 **7(12):** 23–24.

H65 冉崇丕. (2015) 活血止痛汤治疗瘀血型偏头痛 100 例临床观察. 中国民族民间医药 **10:** 45–46.

H66 穆军山. (2007) 养血清脑颗粒治疗偏头痛的临床疗效研究. 福州总医院学报 **Z1:** 106+105.

H67 吴树杰. (2016) 川芎清脑颗粒治疗偏头痛 (风湿蒙蔽, 瘀血阻滞证) 57 例临床研究 (Thesis). 长春中医药大学.

H68 Takaku S, Osono E, Kuribayashi H, *et al.* (2013) A case of migraine without aura that was successfully treated with an herbal medicine. *J Altern Complement Med* **19(12):** 970–972.

6

Pharmacological Actions of Frequently Used Herbs

OVERVIEW

This section reviews the available experimental evidence to explore the possible biological activities and mechanisms of the ten most frequently used Chinese herbs from randomised clinical trials in Chapter 5.

Introduction

As mentioned in Chapter 5, a number of systematic studies have reviewed the potential effects of Chinese herbal medicine (CHM) for migraine symptoms with some promising results found. The evidence from clinical studies included in Chapter 5 has also shown great benefits of CHM in reducing physical and psychological symptoms of migraine. If such treatments play a role in clinical management of migraine, it is important to examine how CHM exerts its clinical effects. This chapter reviews experimental evidence from *in vitro* experimental cells and *in vivo* animal models for some of the most frequently used herbs in clinical trials.

The pathological processes and mechanisms of migraine are complicated and have been described in Chapter 1. The activation and sensitisation of cortical spreading depression (CSD) and trigeminovascular system (TVS), and the decreased regional cerebral blood flow (rCBF) are the key factors contributing to the progression of migraine. Stress and poor sleep quality are the common triggers for migraine.

Animal models of human migraine are vital experimental tools to investigate and assess the therapeutic effects of the herbs and/or compounds on migraine and underlying mechanisms. Various animal models of migraine have been well established. Among of them, nitroglycerin (NTG)-induced migraine and reserpine-induced migraine rodent models are frequently used in experimental studies of migraine. Following NTG (a nitric oxide [NO] donor) injection in rats, the TVS becomes activated to induce hyperalgesia or migraine-like painful and non-painful behaviour.[1] In reserpine-induced migraine rodent models, reserpine (a monoamine-depleting agent) could irreversibly and non-selectively block the vesicular monoamine transporter causing migraine.[2]

Methods

The key herbs reviewed were *chuan xiong* 川芎, *bai zhi* 白芷, *bai shao* 白芍, *dang gui* 当归, *tian ma* 天麻, *xi xin* 细辛, *quan xie* 全蝎, *tao ren* 桃仁, *gan cao* 甘草 and *chai hu* 柴胡. To identify experimental studies and the pharmacological actions of relevance to migraine, the activities of each herb and/or main compounds were examined to identify their therapeutic effects on relieving pains (such as migraine, neuropathic pain and inflammatory pain), attenuating neuroinflammation (such as in microglial cells and astrocytes *in vitro* and neuron-related inflammatory animals) and improving sleep quality (such as sedative and hypnotic effects).

The constituent compounds were identified by searching herbal monographs, high-quality reviews of CHM, materia medica and PubMed. To identify pre-clinical studies, a literature search in PubMed, Google Scholar and PubMed Central was undertaken. Search terms included the scientific names of the plant as well as the Chinese *pinyin*, and names of main compounds found in the plants. These were combined with terms for migraine, analgesia, neuropathic pain, trigeminocervical complex (TCC), cortical oligemia, CSD, neuroinflammation, sedative and hypnotic effects, and migraine rodent models.

Experimental Studies on *Chuan Xiong* 川芎

Chuan xiong 川芎 (*Ligusticum chuanxiong* Hort) belongs to the Umbelliferae family and is used for the treatment of migraine and various cardiovascular and cerebrovascular diseases. So far, more than 200 compounds have been isolated and identified from *L. chuanxiong* and can be grouped into five basic types: volatile oil, phenols and organic acids, alkaloids, phthalides and polysaccharides. Ferulic acid (FA), ligustilide, tetramethylpyrazine (TMP, also known as ligustrazine) and senkyunolide A are the main active constituents of *L. chuanxiong*.[3–5] These compounds demonstrate a broad therapeutic capacity, including effects on cardiovascular and cerebrovascular diseases, as well as antioxidation, anti-inflammation and antidiabetic properties.[3–5] Other pharmacological effects in relation to migraine are discussed.

Anti-migraine Actions

Changes of neurotransmitters and metabolites such as serotonin 5-hydroxytryptamine (5-HT), 5-hydroxytryptophan (5-HTP), 5-hydroxyindoleacetic acid (5-HIAA), norepinephrine (NE) and dopamine (DA) in the central nervous system (CNS) are closely related with the pathogenesis of migraine.[6] In addition, calcitonin gene–related peptide (CGRP), synthesised in the trigeminal ganglion, has been proven to be involved in peripheral neurogenic inflammation and the central sensitisation of migraines.[7]

A great number of *ex vivo* and/or *in vivo* studies demonstrated that the anti-migraine effects of *L. chuanxiong* could be attributed to its various bioactive compounds.

It has been reported that TMP showed antinociceptive effects with elevation of the threshold of thermal nociception in rats.[8] The volatile oil increased the pain threshold induced by a hot plate in mice and in hot radiation-induced headache in rabbits with the inhibition of the expression of the c-fos gene and the secretion of CGRP. This also saw an improvement of 5-HT and endothelin (ET) in plasma in NTG-induced migraine rats.[9] This volatile oil was also demonstrated to have faster onset of action and better analgesic efficacy after nasal administration than oral administration.[10]

Senkyunolide I (SEI), a primary metabolite of ligustilide, has been reported to display anti-migraine effects as it was detectable in both rat plasma and cerebrospinal fluid after oral administration with the ethanol extract of *L. chuanxiong*.[11] The detailed mechanisms of the anti-migraine activity of SEI were explored in NTG-induced migraine rats. The SEI significantly elevated hot plate-induced pain thresholds and reduced acetic acid-induced number of abnormal writhing responses. This was accompanied with improvement of neurotransmitter levels including 5-HT, 5-HTP, 5-HIAA, NE, DA, monoamine turnover rates (5-HT/5-HTP, 5-HIAA/5-HT, and NE/DA), and the reduction of NO in the plasma and whole brain, suggesting that pain relief in migraine model rats might be associated with the levels of monoamine neurotransmitters and their turnover rates and NO levels in the blood and brain.[12] Furthermore, the absorption intensity of SEI and senkyunolide H was observed to be higher in migraine model rats than normal rats, indicating that SEI and senkyunolide H could be two important active ingredients in *L. chuanxiong* for treating migraine.[13] More recently, total alkaloids (TAs) from *L. chuanxiong* were comprehensively evaluated for its anti-migraine effects in both NTG-induced migraine model in rats and reserpine-induced migraine model in mice. Pre-treatment of TAs could upregulate the levels of 5-HT and 5-HIAA in the brain tissue, improve the activation of 5-HT$_{1B}$ receptors and attenuate the activation of c-Jun neurons. The evidence revealed that the TAs not only played a role in preventive efforts in NTG-induced migraine rats, but also offered therapeutic effects in reserpine-induced migraine mice via effects on the function of the endogenous pain modulatory system primarily via the activation of monoamine neurotransmitter 5-HT$_{1B}$ receptor.[14]

In addition to the changes of neurotransmitters in the CNS, activation of the TCC which can cause the development of central sensitisation is also closely related to the pathogenesis of migraine. Effect of TMP on nociceptive trigeminovascular neurotransmission in an *in vivo* rodent model of trigeminovascular dural nociception has demonstrated that TMP could inhibit nociceptive dural-evoked neuronal firing by causing a dose-related inhibition of stimulus-evoked Aδ-fiber responses in the TCC.[15]

Anti-neuroinflammatory Actions

Neuroinflammation is one of the major triggers for migraine. Microglial cells are resident macrophages of the CNS. Activation of microglia and subsequent release of inflammatory mediators, such as NO, tumour necrosis factor α (TNF-α), interleukin-1β (IL-1β), IL-6, interferon-γ (IFN-γ), inducible protein-10 (IP-10) and reactive oxidants, contribute to neuronal inflammation.[16,17] The BV-2 murine microglial cell line is always used as a model of neuroinflammation.

The overall anti-inflammation activity of *L. chuanxiong* has been largely studied.[3–5] However, specific anti-neuroinflammatory activity related to migraine was merely reported. Senkyunolide A and *Z*-ligustilide were found to inhibit the production of proinflammatory mediators in lipopolysaccharide (LPS)-stimulated BV-2 cells. Both compounds could protect neuro-2a cells from neuroinflammatory toxicity induced by the conditioned culture media produced by LPS-stimulated BV-2 cells.[18] Moreover, TMP was also shown to significantly improve the maintenance of chronic constrictive injury (CCI)-induced neuroinflammation and neuropathic pain by suppressing the expression of matrix metalloproteinase-2 and -9 (MMP-2, MMP-9), and phosphorylation of c-Jun N-terminal kinase (JNK) via factor-β-activated kinase 1 (TAK1) signalling pathway in astrocytes.[19]

Sedative Actions

Sleep disturbance is also one of major triggers for migraine and good sleep helps many patients with migraine. It was reported that volatile oil demonstrated to have sedative efficacy after intranasal administration in sodium pentobarbital-induced sleep mice by prolonging the sleeping time, reducing the latency of falling asleep and increasing the rate of sleep onset.[10]

Experimental Studies on *Bai Zhi* 白芷

Bai zhi 白芷 (*Angelicae dahuricae Radix*), belonging to the family Apiaceae, has traditionally been used as an analgesic agent for the treatment of headache caused by the common cold, asthma, coryza and hypertension.[20,21] The bioactive components mainly contain coumarins, volatile oils, polysaccharides and trace elements. Coumarins are the major chemical constituents of *A. dahuricae* roots. *A. dahuricae Radix* has excellent multidirectional pharmacological effects, including anti-inflammatory, antioxidant, antibacterial, antitumour and analgesic activities.[20,21] Other pharmacological effects in relation to migraine are discussed.

Anti-migraine Actions

The essential oil extracted from *A. dahuricae Radix* significantly ameliorated NTG-induced migraine-like symptoms in rats such as irritability, head shaking, frequent scratching of the head by forelimbs, and hind leg shooting of the face. This was accompanied with decreased serum and brain NO and plasma CGRP levels, increased ET levels, and restoration of NTG-induced decreases in the ET/NO ratio.[22]

In addition, it has been reported that *A. dahuricae* could reinforce the anti-migraine activity of other herbs. The total coumarins and volatile oil from *A. dahuricae* could enhance the analgesic effect of corydalis alkaloid (CA) from the root of *Corydalis yanhusuo* through improvement of the plasma concentration of Dl-tetrahydropalmatine.[23] This synergic action of *A. dahuricae* further confirmed that the total coumarins could reinforce the anti-migraine activity of ligustrazine by significantly declining plasma CGRP and serum NO, and increasing plasma ET levels in rats.[24]

Anti-neuroinflammatory Actions

A study clearly demonstrated that *A. dahuricae Radix* could relieve neuropathic pain by suppressing inflammatory mediators. The methanol extract of *A. dahuricae Radix* exhibited dose-dependent antinociceptive and anti-inflammatory effects by improving the acetic acid-induced writhing response and vascular permeability, carrageenan-induced paw oedema, and myeloperoxidase (MPO) activity through inhibition of nitric oxide synthase (iNOS) and NO.[25] Furthermore, *A. dahuricae Radix* could significantly alleviate the LPS-induced increases in the levels of TNF-α, IL-1β, IL-6, iNOS and cyclooxygenase-2 (COX-2) in microglial cells *in vitro* and after spinal cord injury (SCI) *in vivo*.[26] Moreover, when in combination with acetaminophen, a well-known COX-2 selective inhibitor used as an analgesic drug, *A. dahurica* could exert additive or synergistic anti-inflammatory effects in microglia cells.[27]

Sedative Actions

Gamma-aminobutyric acid (GABA) acts as an inhibitory neurotransmitter in the brain and plays a major role in sleep regulation. The GABA$_A$-benzodiazepines (BZD) receptor is considered the most important target for the development of sedative-hypnotic drugs.[28]

Coumarins were reported to possess GABAergic activity. The methanol extracts of *A. dahuricae* were observed to suppress the activities of GABA degradative enzymes such as GABA transaminase (GABA-T) *in vitro*. Of eight isolated coumarins, imperatorin and falcarindiol were found to inhibit GABA-T activities.[29] Furthermore, the benzodiazepine-binding activities of imperatorin and phellopterin were confirmed, suggesting that coumarins possessed the sedative effect for the treatment of insomnia.[30]

Experimental Studies on *Bai Shao* 白芍

Bai shao 白芍 (white peony) is mainly derived from the dried root without bark of *P. lactiflora* Pall. The main characteristic constituents of *P. lactiflora* contain monoterpenoids, triterpenoids, flavonoids, phenols and tannins. Paeoniflorin (PF) is the most abundant (>90%), accounting for the pharmacological activities.[31,32] These compounds have shown multifunctional actions with anti-inflammatory, antioxidant, antiviral, antibacterial, antifungal, antitumour, anti-arthritis, anticoagulant, antiplatelet and immunomodulatory activity.[31,32] Other pharmacological effects in relation to migraine are discussed.

Anti-migraine Actions

Pre-treatment with *P. lactiflora* could not only improve the abnormal behaviours induced by NTG on exploratory, locomotor, freezing, resting and grooming behaviours, but also light-aversive behaviour, spontaneous tactile allodynia, and total travelling distance in the open field test as well. These improvements were accompanied with reduced c-fos and CGRP, indicating that the decrease of c-fos and CGRP played a partial role in the alleviation of migraine related to *P. lactiflora* treatment.[33]

Analgesic Actions

Paeoniflorin has attracted more attention for its antinociceptive activities. Paeoniflorin demonstrated dose-related antinociception on formalin tests in mice. This PF-induced antinociception could be blocked and reversed by Naloxone, nor-binaltorphimine and N(ω)-nitro-L-arginine methyl ester (L-NAME), but could not be potentiated by L-arginine or antagonised by beta-funaltrexamine and ryanodine, indicating that central PF-induced antinociception might be mediated by the activation of kappa-opioid receptor.[34] Other mechanisms of PF-induced antinociception were discovered through adenosine A1 receptor[35] and an interaction with N-methyl-D-aspartate (NMDA) receptors.[36] In addition to PF, albiflorin (AF) also showed analgesic activity. In AF-treated mice, the reduced activation of calmodulin-dependent protein kinase II and JNK in the hypothalamus was believed to contribute to the antinociceptive activity of AF.[37]

Anti-neuroinflammatory Actions

A great number of *in vitro* and/or *in vivo* studies demonstrated that crude extracts and/or compounds of *P. lactiflora* possess strong anti-neuroinflammatory effects. Paeoniflorin significantly blocked LPS-induced hippocampal cell death and productions of NO and IL-1β in hippocampal slice cultures and in microglial cells.[38] Moreover, in morphine-induced robust BV-2 cell activation, PF inhibited the increases of p38 MAP Kinase (MAPK) phosphorylation, nuclear factor kappa-light-chain-enhancer of activated B cells (NF-κB) translocation and proinflammatory cytokine expression. Co-administration of PF with morphine not only enhanced morphine antinociception, but also suppressed morphine-induced expression of toll-like receptor-4 (TLR-4) in both BV-2 cells and the spinal cord of rats.[39] Furthermore, in IFN-α-induced neuroinflammation, PF reversed the abnormal levels of IL-6, IL-1β, IL-9, IL-10, IL-12 and TNF-α by influencing activation of microglia or astrocytes.[40] More recently, PF was reported to mimic apoptosis signal-regulating kinase 1 (ASK1) inhibitor, NQDI1, by reducing the expression of p38 and p-JNK and attenuating neuropathic pain in CCI rats.[41]

Sedative Actions

Administration of *P. lactiflora* was shown to improve sleep quality and coordinate the hypnosis of pentobarbital sodium by inhibiting the CNS and parasympathetic nerve in male Institute of Cancer Research (ICR) mice.[42] Similar sedative and hypnotic effects were observed in PF by decreasing sleeping latency of mice and prolonging sleeping time induced by pentobarbital sodium through modulation of sleep by the 5-HT system in the brain.[43]

Experimental Studies on *Dang Gui* 当归

Dang gui 当归 *(Radix Angelica sinensis)* consists of over 70 compounds. Ferulic acid, *Z*-ligustilide, butylidenephthalide, butylphthalide and polysaccharide are thought to be the main active components in *A. sinensis*.[44,45] These compounds have diverse biological activities, including anti-inflammatory, antioxidant, anti-artherosclerosis, antithrombotic, antiplatelet, antihepatotoxic, anticardiovascular, and immunomodulatory activity.[44,45] Other phar-macological effects in relation to migraine are discussed.

Analgesic Actions

A water extract of *A. sinensis.* possessed significant analgesic activity by decreasing the acetic acid-induced frequency of wringing reac-tion and increasing the pain threshold in the hot-plate procedure in mice.[46] A study suggested that sodium ferulate blocked the initiation of pain and primary afferent sensitisation in the CCI rats.[47] Moreover, FA was shown to not only reverse the reserpine-induced decreases in nociceptive threshold in thermal hyperalgesia and mechanical allo-dynia, but also reverse the decreased NE, 5-HT and DA levels in the brain, suggesting that the effects of FA on reserpine-induced pain occur through modulation of the monoaminergic system.[48] The study was further extended to CCI-induced neuropathic pain by the same research group.[49]

Anti-neuroinflammatory Actions

Pre-treatment with angelica polysaccharide was reported to alleviate LPS-induced inflammation and apoptosis in rat pheochromocytoma PC12 neurons by reducing the expression of IL-1β, IL-6, IL-8, TNF-α and COX-1 through the PI3K/AKT pathway.[50]

Sedative Actions

The $GABA_A$-BZD receptor is considered the most important target for the development of sedative-hypnotic drugs. The water extracts of *A. sinensis* were reported to have high affinity on GABA sites and moderate affinity on 5-HT_{1A} receptors.[51] Furthermore, five fractiona-tions from *A. sinensis* demonstrated competitive binding activity with inhibitory effects on [^{3}H] lysergic acid diethylamide (LSD) binding to the 5-HT_7 receptors, indicating that these compounds might partially contribute to the serotonergic activity of *A. sinensis.*[52]

Experimental Studies on *Tian Ma* 天麻

Tian ma 天麻 (the dried rhizome of *Gastrodia elata*), belongs to the Orchidaceae family and is widely used to treat headache, dizziness, spasm, epilepsy, stoke, amnesia and other disorders. So far, over 81 compounds have been isolated from *G. elata* including phenolics, polysaccharides, organic acids and sterols.[53,54] Gastrodin has been used as the phytochemical marker for the quality control of *G. elata*. Its crude extracts and active compounds have excellent multidirectional effects, including anti-inflammatory, antioxidative, anti-ageing, antitumour, antiepileptic, anticonvulsive, antianxietic, antipsychotic, and neuroprotective effects.[53,54] Other pharmacological effects in relation to migraine are discussed.

Anti-migraine Actions

Acid-sensing ion channels (ASICs), a family of proton-gated cation channels and believed to mediate extracellular acidification-induced pain, have been seen as a novel therapeutic target for migraine with aura.[55] Gastrodin was reported to dose-dependently inhibit proton-gated currents mediated by ASICs in rat dorsal root ganglion neurons, alter acid-evoked membrane excitability and relieve acetic acid-evoked pain in rats. This indicates that inhibition of the activity of ASICs by gastrodin plays a role in reducing aura and headache.[56] Additionally, the effects of gastrodin preventives on nociceptive trigeminovascular neurotransmission in an *in vivo* rodent model of trigeminovascular dural nociception have demonstrated that gastrodin inhibited nociceptive dural-evoked neuronal firing by suppressing ongoing spontaneous activity in the TCC and causing a dose-related inhibition of stimulus-evoked Aδ-fiber responses in the TCC.[15]

Anti-neuroinflammatory Actions

Many studies have demonstrated that *G. elata* ameliorated neuroinflammatory responses. In rat models of kainic acid (KA)-induced epilepsy, treatment with *G. elata* reduced the number of activated microglial cells.[57] In LPS-activated microglial cells, ethanol extract of *G. elata* suppressed TNF-α and IL-1β, and downregulated c-JNK and NF-κB signalling pathways. Further studies verified that 4-hydroxybenzyl alcohol (4-HBA) from *G. elata* might be responsible for anti-neuroinflammatory effects.[58] Moreover, gastrodin significantly attenuated the expression levels of iNOS, COX-2, TNF-α and IL-1β in the LPS-activated microglial cells accompanied with attenuation of expression levels of NF-κB/RelA, phosphorylation of IkB-a, CREB and MAPKs. This indicates that gastrodin might be related to the inhibition of the NF-κB signalling pathway and phosphorylation of MAPKs.[59] This finding was recently confirmed in activated microglia.[60]

Sedative Actions

Aqueous extract of the rhizome of *G. elata* along with its phenolic constituents, 4-hydroxybenzyl alcohol (HA) and 4-hyroxybenzaldehyde (HD), have demonstrated to exert the anxiolytic and myorelaxant effects in mice through 5-HT_{1A} and GABA_A receptors.[61] Moreover, an *in vivo* study showed that ethanol extract of *G. elata* inhibited locomotor activity, prolonged total sleep time, increased rapid eye movement (REM) and reduced sleep latency in pentobarbital-treated mice. *In vitro* studies disclosed that *G. elata* increased intracellular chloride level in primary cultured cerebellar granule cells, accompanied by the increase in expressions of glutamine acid decarboxylase (GAD) and GABAA receptors, suggesting the sedative effect by *G. elata* via the activation of GABA_A-ergic transmission in rodents.[62] Additionally, two active ingredients, N6-(4-hydroxybenzyl) adenine riboside (NHBA) and its analogue N6-(3-methoxyl-4-hydroxybenzyl) adenineriboside (B2) isolated from *G. elata*, were reported to have significant sedative and hypnotic effects through the activation of adenosine A1/A2A receptors[63] and increased GABA levels in the mouse hypothalamus and cortex.[64]

Experimental Studies on *Xi Xin* 细辛

Xi xin 细辛 (Asari/Asiasari Radix et Rhizoma of *Asarum hetero-tropoides* Fr. Schmidt *var. mandshuricum* (Maxim.) Kitag., *A. sieboldii* Miq. *var. seoulense* Nakai and *A. sieboldii* Miq) has been tradition-ally used for alleviating pain, dispelling cold-wind, warming the lungs and resolving accumulated fluids.[65] Major constituents identi-fied from Asari Radix (AR) include volatile oil, lignans, amides, terpenes, flavones, benzene derivatives, apinene, b-pinene, asarinine estragole, eucarvone, kakuol, safrole and methyl eugenol, which exert their anti-inflammatory, antitussive, antitumour, anaesthetic, antinociceptive, antiepileptic, hypothermic and myorelaxant proper-ties.[65] Other pharmacological effects in relation to migraine are discussed.

Analgesic Actions

The crude extracts and pure compounds of AR have traditionally been used to treat pain and inflammation in Asian countries. Administration of methanol extract of AR exerted dramatic antinoci-ceptive effects. Pre-treatment with Naloxone (Nx), a competitive antagonist of μ, κ, and δ opioid receptors, abolished antinociceptive effect of AR, indicating analgesic effects of AR through binding to the μ, κ and δ opioid receptors.[66] Methyleugenol, an essential oil isolated from AR, significantly reduced the duration of formalin-induced lick-ing and biting behaviours similar to diclofenac, an antinociceptive agent.[67] Methyleugenol also inhibited the formalin-induced and NMDA-induced pain-related behaviours similar to muscimol, a $GABA_A$ agonist. However, the antinociception could be suppressed by bicuculline, a $GABA_A$ antagonist, indicating the antinociceptive effect of methyleugenol through inhibition of NMDA receptor-mediated hyperalgesia via GABAA receptors.[67] In addition to methyl-eugenol, orthoeugenol, a synthetic isomer of eugenol, has also been reported to possess the same antinociceptive effects as methyleuge-nol through involvement of the adrenergic system.[68]

Anti-neuroinflammatory Actions

Administration of methanol extract of AR exerted dramatic anti-inflammatory effects, as reflected by inhibiting carrageenan-induced paw oedema similar to ibuprofen, a non-steroidal anti-inflammatory drug.[66] In addition, orthoeugenol demonstrated its anti-inflammatory action as reflected by suppressive effects on vascular permeability in acetic acid-induced peritoneal permeability and leukocyte migration in carrageenan-induced peritonitis. This was accompanied with the subsequent reduction of TNF-α and IL-1β due to inhibition of NF-κB and p38 phosphorylation.[68] Additionally, some volatile oil of AR and non-volatile active components were considered the main effective components contributing to anti-inflammatory activities *in vitro*.[69]

Experimental Studies on *Quan Xie* 全蝎

Quan xie 全蝎 (Scorpion *Buthus martensii* Karsch [BmK]) constitutes a very well-adapted order of predatory animals and has been used for treatment of convulsions and epilepsy in Asia and Africa. Scorpion venom contains a large variety of biologically active components including peptides, enzymes, mucoproteins, free amino acids, nucleotides, lipids, amines, heterocyclic components, inorganic salts and probably other unknown substances.[70–72] These peptides have proven to be effective for the treatment of many conditions including epilepsy, convulsions, facial paralysis, hemiplegia, Parkinson's disease, tumours, pain, and bacterial, malarial, fungal and viral infections, as well as autoimmunity diseases.[70–72] Other pharmacological effects in relation to migraine are discussed.

Analgesic Actions

Sodium channels such as Nav1.3, Nav1.7 and Nav1.8 play important roles in pain pathways. The pain can be attenuated or abolished when these sodium channels are blocked.[73] In recent years, a range of scorpion analgesic peptides has been obtained and proved to target sodium channels.

Buthus martensii Karsch venom containing mixtures of polypeptides showed its remarkable analgesic activities. As a β-anti-excitatory neurotoxin, BmK AS was reported to markedly reduce formalin-evoked biphasic spontaneous nociceptive behaviours in a dose-dependent manner, accompanied with the inhibition of formalin-induced c-fos expression and the sodium currents in a dose-dependent manner. This occurred without affecting the potassium currents or Ca^{2+} influx, suggesting that the remarkable anti-nociceptive effects of BmK AS in both the periphery and spinal cord might be associated with particular targets on sodium channels.[74] It was shown that the subtype of sodium channels, Nav1.3, was responsible for analgesic activity.[75] In addition, anti-neuroexcitation peptide (ANEP),[76] another β-anti-excitatory neurotoxin, and BmNaL-3SS2 and BmKBTx[77] also showed analgesic activity through inhibition of Nav1.7. Additionally, BmK AGAP demonstrated dose-dependent analgesic activity in a mouse inflammatory pain model through an MAPKs-mediated mechanism.[78] More interestedly, unlike the peptides mentioned above which acted on sodium channels, BmK-YA, an amidated peptide containing an enkephalin-like peptide in BmK venom, was reported to interact with μ, δ and κ opioid receptors. It was also demonstrated to be more potent than morphine in terms of analgesic activity through targeting opioid receptors G protein-coupled receptors.[79]

Experimental Studies on *Tao Ren* 桃仁

Tao ren 桃仁 (the fruit-kernel of peach/semen of *Prunus persica* (L.) Batsch and *Prunus davidiana* (Carr.) Franch) belongs to the Rosaceae family and is well known for treatment of hemasthenosis, constipation, chronic rhinitis, cough, asthma, dysmenorrhea, arthritis and diarrhoea. Various compounds have been isolated from semen of *Prunus,* including amygdalin, cyanogenic glycosides, prunasin, emulsion, glycerides and sterols.[80,81] Pharmacological studies have demonstrated that *P. persica* exhibits an antitumour-promoting activity, acetylcholinesterase inhibition, antiallergic, antioxidant and antihepatocellular carcinoma activity.[80,81] Other pharmacological effects in relation to migraine are discussed.

Analgesic Actions

Antinociceptive effects of nectarine kernel alcoholic extract (NAE) were reported on thermally induced analgesia using the hot-plate model in rats and acetic acid-induced writhing reflex in mice. Administration of NAE demonstrated to prolong the reaction time on the hot plate test comparable to the standard drug tramadol. Meanwhile, administration of NAE was also shown to reduce writhing responses in acetic acid-injected mice comparable to the standard drug indomethacin. Furthermore, total polyphenolic and flavonoid identified from NAE were responsible for antinociceptive effects of NAE.[82]

Anti-neuroinflammatory Actions

The acute anti-inflammatory effect of NAE was evaluated by the carrageenan-induced rat hind paw oedema test. Treatment with NAE significantly reduced paw oedema on the both early and late phases compared with indomethacin, a non-steroidal anti-inflammatory drug (NSAID), only on the late phase, indicating the anti-inflammatory effect of NAE was comparable to indomethacin on the late phase, in addition to its effect on the early phase of inflammation.[82]

Experimental Studies on *Gan Cao* 甘草

Gan cao 甘草 (liquorice), originated from three plants: *Glycyrrhiza uralensis* Fisch., *Glycyrrhiza inflata* Bat. and *Glycyrrhiza glabra* L., and has been traditionally used to treat coughs, influenza, gastric ulcers, liver damage and detoxification. At least 400 isolated compounds have been determined. The main bioactive constituents of liquorice are triterpene saponins (more than 20) and various types of flavonoids (more than 300).[83–85] These compounds exhibit extensive pharmacological properties such as anti-inflammatory, antiallergic, antioxidative, antiviral, anticarcinogenic, antithrombotic and antiulceric activities and immunoregulatory, hepatoprotective, and cardioprotective effects.[83–85] Other pharmacological effects in relation to migraine are discussed.

Analgesic Actions

Isoliquiritigenin (ISL), a flavonoid from *G. glabra*, not only demonstrated the analgesic and uterine relaxant effects *in vitro*, but also effective activity in reducing pain in the acetic acid-induced writhing response and hot-plate test *in vivo* through involvement of Ca^{2+} channels, NOS and COX.[86] Liquiritin (LQ) proved its protective efficacy on CCI-induced neuropathic pain in mice by significantly alleviating the CCI-evoked behavioural variations in mechanical allodynia, cold allodynia and thermal hyperalgesia. Moreover, LQ inhibits the activation of glial cells (microglia and astrocyte) by attenuating the CCI-induced overexpression of TNF-α, IL-6 and IL-1β, indicating that the protective effect on neuropathic pain by LQ might be attributed to its anti-inflammatory actions.[87]

Anti-neuroinflammatory Actions

Plenty of *in vitro* and/or *in vivo* studies have demonstrated that crude extracts and/or compounds of liquorice possess strong anti-neuroinflammatory effects. Glabridin, a flavonoid isolated from *G. glabra*, was reported to inhibit microglial activation by blocking DNA-binding activity of NF-κB and Activator protein 1 (AP-1).[88] Glycyrrhizin (GRZ), a triterpenoid saponin from *G. glabra*, demonstrated anti-neuroinflammatory activity in systemic LPS-treated mice through inhibiting proinflammatory cytokines and ionised calcium-binding adaptor molecule 1 (Iba1, a marker of microglial activation in the hippocampal tissue).[89] Additionally, GA, LQ and liquiritigenin (LG) also demonstrated their anti-neuroinflammatory activities in microglial cells.[90] More recently, GA was further confirmed against

LPS-induced neuroinflammation in an LPS-induced Alzheimer's mouse model via inhibiting activation of TLR4 signalling pathways.[91]

Sedative Actions

Ethanol extract of *G. glabra* showed its hypnotic effect on pentobarbital-induced sleep in mice. It dose-dependently decreased sleep latency and increased sleep duration similar to sleep drug diazepam and increased the amount of non-REM sleep without a decrease of delta activity in a way similar to that of physiological sleep. This effect could be completely suppressed by flumazenil, a specific $GABA_A$-BZD receptor antagonist.[92] These findings were further extended to its flavonoid glabrol, indicating *G. glabra*- and glabro-induced sleep through a positive allosteric modulation of $GABA_A$-BZD receptors.[92] Glabridin has shown GABA response similar to zolpidem, a hypnotic drug, implying that the sedative and hypnotic effects of glabridin is largely due to potentiation of GABAergic suppression in dorsal raphe neurons by $GABA_A$ receptor actions.[93]

Experimental Studies on *Chai Hu* 柴胡

Chai hu 柴胡 *(Radix Bupleuri)*, derived from the dried roots of *Bupleurum chinense* DC. and *Bupleurum scorzonerifolium* Wild, has been widely used to treat influenza, fever, chills, chest pain, inflammation, malaria, irregular menstruation, hepatitis, uterine prolapse and rectocele in Asian countries.[94,95] More than 280 compounds have been identified from *Radix Bupleuri*, including triterpenoid saponins, lignins, essential oils, flavones, phenylpropanols, coumarins, polyynes, polyacetylenes and polysaccharides. Saikosaponins A and D are commonly used for quality evaluation of *Radix Bupleuri*.[94,95] These compounds have been extensively studied and show multiple functions with greater potential anti-inflammatory, antioxidant, antiviral, antibacterial, antitumour, anti-arthritis, anticoagulant and antiplatelet, as well as immunomodulatory, activity.[94,95] Other pharmacological effects in relation to migraine are discussed.

Analgesic Actions

Saikosaponin A has been demonstrated to attenuate neuropathic pain induced by mouse sciatic nerve CCI. Administration of saikosaponin reversed CCI-induced mechanical allodynia and thermal hyperalgesia and resulted in the most pain relief through attenuating CCI-increased levels of TNF-a, IL-1β and IL-2, and decreasing expression of p38 MAPK and NF-kB p65 in the spinal cord of CCI rats.[96]

Anti-neuroinflammatory Actions

It was reported that treatment with ethanol extract of *B. falcatum* (BFE) not only significantly inhibited the expression and activation of MMP-2 and MMP-9 after SCI, but also suppressed the expression of inflammatory mediators including TNF-α, IL-1β, COX-2 and iNOS to attenuate neuroinflammation.[97] This finding was further explored in LPS-stimulated microglial cells and LPS-injected mice. *In vitro*, BFE efficiently suppressed the production of LPS-induced NO, iNOS, reactive oxygen species, IL-6, IL-1β, TNF-α, NF-κB p65/RELA mRNA levels and NF-κB-dependent transcription in the nuclei of activated microglial cells. *In vivo*, BFE suppressed the activation of astrocytes and microglia in the brains of LPS-injected mice. Is also blocked the LPS-induced increase in glial fibrillary acidic protein and Iba-1 positive cells in the hippocampus. Similarly, three pure compounds from *B. falcatum*; saikosaponin 3 (SB3), saikosaponin 4 (SB4) and saikosaponin D (SD), displayed the same anti-inflammatory activity as BEF in LPS-stimulated microglial cells. These data indicated that BFE and its bioactive compounds possessed anti-neuroinflammatory effects *in vivo* as well as *in vitro*.[98]

Sedative Actions

As DA, 5-HT and GABA are very important receptors for CNS neurotransmitters, the water extract of *B. falcatum* was reported to have moderate affinity to DA D1 and D2 and 5-HT$_{1A}$ receptors in male ICR mice.[51]

Summary of Pharmacological Actions of the Common Herbs

Each of these ten herbs has attracted research attention in experimental models of relevance to migraine. The special actions of relieving migraine were observed in some of herbs, including *chuan xiong* 川芎, *bai zhi* 白芷, *bai shao* 白芍 and *tian ma* 天麻 through modulation of neurotransmitters such as 5-HT, 5-HTP, 5-HIAA, NE and DA in the CNS and the expression of c-fos and CGRP. In particularly, *chuan xiong* 川芎, *bai zhi* 白芷 and *tian ma* 天麻 exerted very strong anti-migraine effects.

When the studies on anti-migraine activities of herbs were not available, the general analgesic activity was instead searched for the therapeutic effects. Analgesic actions were observed in most of the herbs. With the exception of *tao ren* 桃仁 and *chai hu* 柴胡, all herbs showed very powerful antinociceptive properties through suppressing the expression of inflammatory mediators, inhibiting NMDA receptor-mediated hyperalgesia via GABAA receptors, showing opioid-like activity and modulating sodium channels.

The overall anti-inflammatory effect has been reported in all ten herbs and has been well known to enhance the innate immune system against whole-body inflammation, which in turn is beneficial to brain inflammation as well. Specific anti-neuroinflammatory actions were also observed in all of the herbs, through suppressing the activation of microglial cells and astrocytes and subsequently reducing the release of inflammatory mediators.

The sedative and hypnotic actions were observed in most herbs, particularly in *tian ma* 天麻 and *gan cao* 甘草, through modulating the GABAergic system. In addition, some herbs have been assessed in NTG-induced and/or reserpine-induced migraine rodent models.

These *in vitro* and *in vivo* studies examined herb actions specific to migraine and provide potential explanations of the clinical benefits of all the common herbs. The findings highlight that CHM have multiple components which can act on multiple pathways relevant to migraine. This fully reflects the multiple-target synergy characteristics of Chinese medicine generally.

References

1. Greco R, Ferrigno A, Demartini C, *et al.* (2015) Evaluation of ADMA-DDAH-NOS axis in specific brain areas following nitroglycerin administration: Study in an animal model of migraine. *J Headache Pain* **16:** 560.

2. de Freitas CM, Busanello A, Schaffer LF, *et al.* (2016) Behavioral and neurochemical effects induced by reserpine in mice. *Psychopharmacology (Berl)* **233(3):** 457–467.

3. Chen Z, Zhang C, Gao F, *et al.* (2018) A systematic review on the rhizome of *Ligusticum chuanxiong* Hort. (Chuanxiong). *Food Chem Toxicol* **119:** 309–325.

4. Li W, Tang Y, Chen Y, *et al.* (2012) Advances in the chemical analysis and biological activities of *chuanxiong*. *Molecules* **17(9):** 10614–10651.

5. Ran X, Ma L, Peng C, *et al.* (2011) *Ligusticum chuanxiong* Hort: A review of chemistry and pharmacology. *Pharm Biol* **49(11):** 1180–1189.

6. Viguier F, Michot B, Hamon M, *et al.* (2013) Multiple roles of serotonin in pain control mechanisms: Implications of 5-HT(7) and other 5-HT receptor types. *Eur J Pharmacol* **716(1–3):** 8–16.

7. Edvinsson L. (2017) The trigeminovascular pathway: Role of CGRP and CGRP receptors in migraine. *Headache* **57(Suppl 2):** 47–55.

8. Bie BH, Chen Y, Zhao ZQ. (2006) Ligustrazine inhibits high voltage-gated Ca(2+) and TTX-resistant Na(+) channels of primary sensory neuron and thermal nociception in the rat: A study on peripheral mechanism. *Neurosci Bull* **22(2):** 79–84.

9. Peng C, Xie X, Wang L, *et al.* (2009) Pharmacodynamic action and mechanism of volatile oil from Rhizoma Ligustici Chuanxiong Hort. on treating headache. *Phytomedicine* **16(1):** 25–34.

10. Guo J, Duan JA, Tang Y, *et al.* (2010) Fast onset of action and the analgesic and sedative efficacy of essential oil from Rhizoma Chuanxiong after nasal administration. *Pharmazie* **65(4):** 296–299.

11. Yuan Y, Lin X, Xu DS, *et al.* (2010) *In vivo* transmigration of anti-migrainous compounds from *Ligusticum chuanxiong* Hort. *J Chin Pharm Sci* **45(9):** 694–697.

12. Wang YH, Liang S, Xu DS, *et al.* (2011) Effect and mechanism of senkyunolide I as an anti-migraine compound from *Ligusticum chuanxiong*. *J Pharm Pharmacol* **63(2):** 261–266.

13. Zhao X, Ma T, Zhang C, *et al.* (2015) Simultaneous determination of senkyunolide I and senkyunolide H in rat plasma by LC-MS: Application to a comparative pharmacokinetic study in normal and migrainous rats after oral administration of Chuanxiong Rhizoma extract. *Biomed Chromatogr* **29(9):** 1297–1303.

14. Pu ZH, Peng C, Xie XF, *et al.* (2019) Alkaloids from the rhizomes of *Ligusticum striatum* exert antimigraine effects through regulating 5-HT1B receptor and c-Jun. *J Ethnopharmacol* **237:** 39–46.

15. Zhao Y, Martins-Oliveira M, Akerman S, *et al.* (2018) Comparative effects of traditional Chinese and Western migraine medicines in an animal model of nociceptive trigeminovascular activation. *Cephalalgia* **38(7):** 1215–1224.

16. Biber K, Vinet J, Boddeke HW. (2008) Neuron-microglia signalling: Chemokines as versatile messengers. *J Neuroimmunol* **198(1–2):** 69–74.

17. Lee M. (2013) Neurotransmitters and microglial-mediated neuroinflammation. *Curr Protein Pept Sci* **14(1):** 21–32.

18. Or TC, Yang CL, Law AH, *et al.* (2011) Isolation and identification of anti-inflammatory constituents from *Ligusticum chuanxiong* and their underlying mechanisms of action on microglia. *Neuropharmacology* **60(6):** 823–831.

19. Jiang L, Pan CL, Wang CY, *et al.* (2017) Selective suppression of the JNK-MMP2/9 signal pathway by tetramethylpyrazine attenuates neuropathic pain in rats. *J Neuroinflammation* **14(1):** 174.

20. Qi B, Yang W, Ding N, *et al.* (2019) Pyrrole 2-carbaldehyde derived alkaloids from the roots of *Angelica dahurica. J Nat Med* **73(4):** 769–776.

21. Wang J, Lian P, Yu Q, *et al.* (2017) Purification, characterization and procoagulant activity of polysaccharides from *Angelica dahurice* roots. *Chem Cent J* **11:** 17.

22. Sun J, Li H, Sun J, *et al.* (2017) Chemical composition and antimigraine activity of essential oil of *Angelicae dahuricae* radix. *J Med Food* **20(8):** 797–803.

23. Liao ZG, Liang XL, Zhu JY, *et al.* (2010) Correlation between synergistic action of Radix *Angelica dahurica* extracts on analgesic effects of Corydalis alkaloid and plasma concentration of dl-THP. *J Ethnopharmacol* **129(1):** 115–120.

24. Feng S, He X, Zhong P, *et al.* (2018) A metabolism-based synergy for total coumarin extract of Radix Angelicae Dahuricae and Ligustrazine on migraine treatment in rats. *Molecules* **23(5):** 1004.

25. Kang OH, Chae HS, Oh YC, *et al.* (2008) Anti-nociceptive and anti-inflammatory effects of Angelicae dahuricae radix through inhibition of the expression of inducible nitric oxide synthase and NO production. *Am J Chin Med* **36(5):** 913–928.

26. Moon YJ, Lee JY, Oh MS, *et al.* (2012) Inhibition of inflammation and oxidative stress by Angelica dahuricae radix extract decreases apoptotic cell death and improves functional recovery after spinal cord injury. *J Neurosci Res* **90(1):** 243–256.

27. Kim H, Bae S, Kwon KY, *et al.* (2015) A combinational effect of acetaminophen and oriental herbs on the regulation of inflammatory mediators in microglia cell line, BV2. *Anat Cell Biol* **48(4):** 244–250.

28. Erman MK. (2005) Therapeutic options in the treatment of insomnia. *J Clin Psychiatry* **66(Suppl 9):** 18–23; quiz 42–43.

29. Choi SY, Ahn EM, Song MC, *et al.* (2005) *In vitro* GABA-transaminase inhibitory compounds from the root of *Angelica dahurica*. *Phytother Res* **19(10):** 839–845.

30. Singhuber J, Baburin I, Ecker GF, *et al.* (2011) Insights into structure-activity relationship of GABAA receptor modulating coumarins and furanocoumarins. *Eur J Pharmacol* **668(1–2):** 57–64.

31. He DY, Dai SM. (2011) Anti-inflammatory and immunomodulatory effects of paeonia lactiflora Pall., a traditional chinese herbal medicine. *Front Pharmacol* **2:** 10.

32. Parker S, May B, Zhang C, *et al.* (2016) A pharmacological review of bioactive constituents of *Paeonia lactiflora* Pallas and *Paeonia veitchii* Lynch. *Phytother Res* **30(9):** 1445–1473.

33. Liao CC, Li JM, Chen CH, *et al.* (2019) Effect of Paeonia lactiflora, a traditional Chinese herb, on migraines based on clinical application and animal behavior analyses. *Biomed Pharmacother* **118:** 109276.

34. Tsai HY, Lin YT, Tsai CH, *et al.* (2001) Effects of paeoniflorin on the formalin-induced nociceptive behaviour in mice. *J Ethnopharmacol* **75(2–3):** 267–271.

35. Zhang XJ, Chen HL, Li Z, *et al.* (2009) Analgesic effect of paeoniflorin in rats with neonatal maternal separation-induced visceral hyperalgesia is mediated through adenosine A(1) receptor by inhibiting the extracellular signal-regulated protein kinase (ERK) pathway. *Pharmacol Biochem Behav* **94(1):** 88–97.

36. Chen YF, Lee MM, Fang HL, *et al.* (2016) Paeoniflorin inhibits excitatory amino acid agonist and high-dose morphine-induced nociceptive

behavior in mice via modulation of N-methyl-D-aspartate receptors. *BMC Complement Altern Med* **16:** 240.

37. Zhang Y, Sun D, Meng Q, *et al.* (2016) Calcium channels contribute to albiflorin-mediated antinociceptive effects in mouse model. *Neurosci Lett* **628:** 105–109.

38. Nam KN, Yae CG, Hong JW, *et al.* (2013) Paeoniflorin, a monoterpene glycoside, attenuates lipopolysaccharide-induced neuronal injury and brain microglial inflammatory response. *Biotechnol Lett* **35(8):** 1183–1189.

39. Jiang C, Xu L, Chen L, *et al.* (2015) Selective suppression of microglial activation by paeoniflorin attenuates morphine tolerance. *Eur J Pain* **19(7):** 908–919.

40. Li J, Huang S, Huang W, *et al.* (2017) Paeoniflorin ameliorates interferon-alpha-induced neuroinflammation and depressive-like behaviors in mice. *Oncotarget* **8(5):** 8264–8282.

41. Zhou D, Zhang S, Hu L, *et al.* (2019) Inhibition of apoptosis signal-regulating kinase by paeoniflorin attenuates neuroinflammation and ameliorates neuropathic pain. *J Neuroinflammation* **16(1):** 83.

42. Zhang XF. (2008) Effects of *Paeonia lactiflora* extract on sleep improvement in rats. *Contemp Med* **33:** e4.

43. Li Y, Wu P, Ning Y, *et al.* (2014) Sedative and hypnotic effect of freeze-dried paeoniflorin and sini san freeze-dried powder in pentobarbital sodium-induced mice. *J Tradit Chin Med* **34(2):** 184–187.

44. Chao WW, Lin BF. (2011) Bioactivities of major constituents isolated from *Angelica sinensis* (Danggui). *Chin Med* **6:** 29.

45. Wei WL, Zeng R, Gu CM, *et al.* (2016) Angelica sinensis in China: A review of botanical profile, ethnopharmacology, phytochemistry and chemical analysis. *J Ethnopharmacol* **190:** 116–141.

46. Song M. Li Q, He C. (2009) Identification and analgetic effect of *Angelica sinensis* extract. *Journal of Xianning University* **23:** 194–196.

47. Zhang A, Xu C, Liang S, *et al.* (2008) Role of sodium ferulate in the nociceptive sensory facilitation of neuropathic pain injury mediated by P2X(3) receptor. *Neurochem Int* **53(6–8):** 278–282.

48. Xu Y, Zhang L, Shao T, *et al.* (2013) Ferulic acid increases pain threshold and ameliorates depression-like behaviors in reserpine-treated mice: Behavioral and neurobiological analyses. *Metab Brain Dis* **28(4):** 571–583.

49. Xu Y, Lin D, Yu X, *et al.* (2016) The antinociceptive effects of ferulic acid on neuropathic pain: Involvement of descending monoaminergic system and opioid receptors. *Oncotarget* **7(15):** 20455–20468.

50. Xie Y, Zhang H, Zhang Y, *et al.* (2018) Chinese Angelica polysaccharide (CAP) alleviates LPS-Induced inflammation and apoptosis by down-regulating COX-1 in PC12 Cells. *Cell Physiol Biochem* **49(4):** 1380–1388.

51. Liao JF, Jan YM, Huang SY, *et al.* (1995) Evaluation with receptor binding assay on the water extracts of ten CNS-active Chinese herbal drugs. *Proc Natl Sci Counc Repub China B* **19(3):** 151–158.

52. Deng S, Chen SN, Yao P, *et al.* (2006) Serotonergic activity-guided phytochemical investigation of the roots of *Angelica sinensis*. *J Nat Prod* **69(4):** 536–541.

53. Liu Y, Gao J, Peng M, *et al.* (2018) A review on central nervous system effects of gastrodin. *Front Pharmacol* **9:** 24.

54. Zhan HD, Zhou HY, Sui YP, *et al.* (2016) The rhizome of Gastrodia elata Blume: An ethnopharmacological review. *J Ethnopharmacol* **189:** 361–385.

55. Holland PR, Akerman S, Andreou AP, *et al.* (2012) Acid-sensing ion channel 1: A novel therapeutic target for migraine with aura. *Ann Neurol* **72(4):** 559–563.

56. Qiu F, Liu TT, Qu ZW, *et al.* (2014) Gastrodin inhibits the activity of acid-sensing ion channels in rat primary sensory neurons. *Eur J Pharmacol* **731:** 50–57.

57. Hsieh CL, Chen CL, Tang NY, *et al.* (2005) Gastrodia elata BL mediates the suppression of nNOS and microglia activation to protect against neuronal damage in kainic acid-treated rats. *Am J Chin Med* **33(4):** 599–611.

58. Kim BW, Koppula S, Kim JW, *et al.* (2012) Modulation of LPS-stimulated neuroinflammation in BV-2 microglia by Gastrodia elata: 4-hydroxybenzyl alcohol is the bioactive candidate. *J Ethnopharmacol* **139(2):** 549–557.

59. Dai JN, Zong Y, Zhong LM, *et al.* (2011) Gastrodin inhibits expression of inducible NO synthase, cyclooxygenase-2 and proinflammatory cytokines in cultured LPS-stimulated microglia via MAPK pathways. *PLoS One* **6(7):** e21891.

60. Li JJ, Liu SJ, Liu XY, *et al.* (2018) Herbal compounds with special reference to gastrodin as potential therapeutic agents for microglia mediated neuroinflammation. *Curr Med Chem* **25(42):** 5958–5974.

61. Jung JW, Yoon BH, Oh HR, *et al.* (2006) Anxiolytic-like effects of *Gastrodia elata* and its phenolic constituents in mice. *Biol Pharm Bull* **29(2):** 261–265.

62. Choi JJ, Oh EH, Lee MK, *et al.* (2014) Gastrodiae rhizoma ethanol extract enhances pentobarbital-induced sleeping behaviors and rapid eye movement sleep via the activation of GABA A-ergic transmission in rodents. *Evid Based Complement Alternat Med* **2014:** 426843.

63. Zhang Y, Li M, Kang RX, *et al.* (2012) NHBA isolated from *Gastrodia elata* exerts sedative and hypnotic effects in sodium pentobarbital-treated mice. *Pharmacol Biochem Behav* **102(3):** 450–457.

64. Shi Y, Dong JW, Tang LN, *et al.* (2014) N(6)-(3-methoxyl-4-hydroxybenzyl) adenine riboside induces sedative and hypnotic effects via GAD enzyme activation in mice. *Pharmacol Biochem Behav* **126:** 146–151.

65. Drew AK, Whyte IM, Bensoussan A, *et al.* (2002) Chinese herbal medicine toxicology database: Monograph on Herba Asari, "xi xin". *J Toxicol Clin Toxicol* **40(2):** 169–172.

66. Kim SJ, Gao Zhang C, Taek Lim J. (2003) Mechanism of anti-nociceptive effects of Asarum sieboldii Miq. radix: Potential role of bradykinin, histamine and opioid receptor-mediated pathways. *J Ethnopharmacol* **88(1):** 5–9.

67. Yano S, Suzuki Y, Yuzurihara M, *et al.* (2006) Antinociceptive effect of methyleugenol on formalin-induced hyperalgesia in mice. *Eur J Pharmacol* **553(1–3):** 99–103.

68. Fonseca DV, Salgado PR, Aragao Neto Hde C, *et al.* (2016) Ortho-eugenol exhibits anti-nociceptive and anti-inflammatory activities. *Int Immunopharmacol* **38:** 402–408.

69. Jing Y, Zhang YF, Shang MY, *et al.* (2017) Chemical constituents from the roots and rhizomes of *Asarum heterotropoides* var. *mandshuricum* and the *in vitro* anti-inflammatory activity. *Molecules* **22(1):** 125.

70. Cao Z, Di Z, Wu Y, *et al.* (2014) Overview of scorpion species from China and their toxins. *Toxins (Basel)* **6(3):** 796–815.

71. Li Z, Hu P, Wu W, *et al.* (2019) Peptides with therapeutic potential in the venom of the scorpion *Buthus martensii* Karsch. *Peptides* **115:** 43–50.

72. Ortiz E, Gurrola GB, Schwartz EF, *et al.* (2015) Scorpion venom components as potential candidates for drug development. *Toxicon* **93:** 125–135.

73. Wood JN, Boorman JP, Okuse K, *et al.* (2004) Voltage-gated sodium channels and pain pathways. *J Neurobiol* **61(1):** 55–71.

74. Liu T, Pang XY, Jiang F, *et al.* (2008) Anti-nociceptive effects induced by intrathecal injection of BmK AS, a polypeptide from the venom of

Chinese-scorpion *Buthus martensi* Karsch, in rat formalin test. *J Ethnopharmacol* **117(2):** 332–338.

75. Liu ZR, Tao J, Dong BQ, *et al.* (2012) Pharmacological kinetics of BmK AS, a sodium channel site 4-specific modulator on Nav1.3. *Neurosci Bull* **28(3):** 209–221.

76. Song Y, Liu Z, Zhang Q, *et al.* (2017) Investigation of binding modes and functional surface of scorpion toxins ANEP to sodium channels 1.7. *Toxins (Basel)* **9(12):** 387.

77. Lin S, Wang X, Hu X, *et al.* (2017) Recombinant expression, functional characterization of two scorpion venom toxins with three disulfide bridges from the chinese scorpion *Buthus martensii* Karsch. *Protein Pept Lett* **24(3):** 235–240.

78. Mao Q, Ruan J, Cai X, *et al.* (2013) Antinociceptive effects of analgesic-antitumor peptide (AGAP), a neurotoxin from the scorpion *Buthus martensii* Karsch, on formalin-induced inflammatory pain through a mitogen-activated protein kinases-dependent mechanism in mice. *PLoS One* **8(11):** e78239.

79. Zhang Y, Xu J, Wang Z, *et al.* (2012) BmK-YA, an enkephalin-like peptide in scorpion venom. *PLoS One* **7(7):** e40417.

80. Aziz S, Habib-ur Rahman. (2013) Biological activities of *Prunus persica* L. batch. *J Med Plants Res* **7:** 947–951.

81. Fukuda T, Ito H, Mukainaka T, *et al.* (2003) Anti-tumor promoting effect of glycosides from *Prunus persica* seeds. *Biol Pharm Bull* **26(2):** 271–273.

82. Elshamy AI, Abdallah HMI, El Gendy AEG, *et al.* (2019) Evaluation of anti-inflammatory, antinociceptive, and antipyretic activities of *Prunus persica* var. *nucipersica* (nectarine) kernel. *Planta Med* **85(11–12):** 1016–1023.

83. Asl MN, Hosseinzadeh H. (2008) Review of pharmacological effects of Glycyrrhiza sp. and its bioactive compounds. *Phytother Res* **22(6):** 709–724.

84. Ji S, Li Z, Song W, *et al.* (2016) Bioactive constituents of *Glycyrrhiza uralensis* (liquorice): Discovery of the effective components of a traditional herbal medicine. *J Nat Prod* **79(2):** 281–292.

85. Zhang Q, Ye M. (2009) Chemical analysis of the Chinese herbal medicine Gan-Cao (liquorice). *J Chromatogr A* **1216(11):** 1954–1969.

86. Shi Y, Wu D, Sun Z, *et al.* (2012) Analgesic and uterine relaxant effects of isoliquiritigenin, a flavone from *Glycyrrhiza glabra*. *Phytother Res* **26(9):** 1410–1417.

87. Zhang MT, Wang B, Jia YN, *et al.* (2017) Neuroprotective effect of liquiritin against neuropathic pain induced by chronic constriction injury of the sciatic nerve in mice. *Biomed Pharmacother* **95**: 186–198.

88. Park SH, Kang JS, Yoon YD, *et al.* (2010) Glabridin inhibits lipopolysaccharide-induced activation of a microglial cell line, BV-2, by blocking NF-kappaB and AP-1. *Phytother Res* **24 (Suppl 1)**: S29–S34.

89. Song JH, Lee JW, Shim B, *et al.* (2013) Glycyrrhizin alleviates neuroinflammation and memory deficit induced by systemic lipopolysaccharide treatment in mice. *Molecules* **18(12)**: 15788–15803.

90. Yu JY, Ha JY, Kim KM, *et al.* (2015) Anti-Inflammatory activities of liquorice extract and its active compounds, glycyrrhizic acid, liquiritin and liquiritigenin, in BV2 cells and mice liver. *Molecules* **20(7)**: 13041–13054.

91. Liu W, Huang S, Li Y, *et al.* (2019) Suppressive effect of glycyrrhizic acid against lipopolysaccharide-induced neuroinflammation and cognitive impairment in C57 mice via toll-like receptor 4 signalling pathway. *Food Nutr Res*: **63**.

92. Cho S, Park JH, Pae AN, *et al.* (2012) Hypnotic effects and GABAergic mechanism of liquorice (*Glycyrrhiza glabra*) ethanol extract and its major flavonoid constituent glabrol. *Bioorg Med Chem* **20(11)**: 3493–3501.

93. Jin Z, Kim S, Cho S, *et al.* (2013) Potentiating effect of glabridin on GABAA receptor-mediated responses in dorsal raphe neurons. *Planta Med* **79(15)**: 1408–1412.

94. Sun P, Li Y, Wei S, *et al.* (2019) Pharmacological effects and chemical constituents of Bupleurum. *Mini Rev Med Chem* **19(1)**: 34–55.

95. Yang F, Dong X, Yin X, *et al.* (2017) Radix Bupleuri: A review of traditional uses, botany, phytochemistry, pharmacology, and toxicology. *Biomed Res Int* **2017**: 7597596.

96. Zhou X, Cheng H, Xu D, *et al.* (2014) Attenuation of neuropathic pain by saikosaponin a in a rat model of chronic constriction injury. *Neurochem Res* **39(11)**: 2136–2142.

97. Lee JY, Kim HS, Oh TH, *et al.* (2010) Ethanol extract of *Bupleurum falcatum* improves functional recovery by inhibiting matrix metalloproteinases-2 and -9 activation and inflammation after spinal cord injury. *Exp Neurobiol* **19(3)**: 146–154.

98. Park WH, Kang S, Piao Y, *et al.* (2015) Ethanol extract of *Bupleurum falcatum* and saikosaponins inhibit neuroinflammation via inhibition of NF-kappaB. *J Ethnopharmacol* **174**: 37–44.

7

Clinical Evidence for Acupuncture and Other Chinese Medicine Therapy

OVERVIEW

Acupuncture is commonly used in clinical practice for the management of migraine. Other Chinese medicine therapies are also recommended in clinical guidelines. This chapter evaluates the available clinical evidence of acupuncture and other Chinese medicine therapies for migraine. Where appropriate, data are pooled in meta-analyses to assess their overall effects for different outcome measures. The quality of evidence is also evaluated to assess the strength of available data. Frequently used acupuncture points are summarised. Through the rigorous selection process, 50 clinical studies of acupuncture therapies were included in the evaluation, without any studies of other Chinese medicine therapy being included.

Introduction

Acupuncture therapies are recommended in clinical guidelines and commonly used in clinical practice for the management of migraine. Other Chinese medicine (CM) therapies, such as *tuina* 推拿 therapy and moxibustion, are also recommended in clinical guidelines. A rigorous screening process was undertaken to identify previously published systematic reviews and clinical studies of these therapies for the treatment of migraine. The clinical studies included randomised controlled trials (RCTs), non-randomised controlled clinical trials (CCTs) and non-controlled studies. As in Chapter 5, the evidence from RCTs has been pooled for evaluation of the efficacy and safety of acupuncture alone, or in combination with conventional therapy for episodic migraine. The CCTs were evaluated using the same approach as for RCTs and are described separately. Evidence from non-controlled studies is more difficult to evaluate; therefore the approach was taken to describe the characteristics of the study, details of the intervention and any adverse events (AEs). The findings of the literature search are presented in this chapter.

Through the rigorous selection process, 50 clinical studies of acupuncture therapies were included in the evaluation, without any studies of other CM therapy being included.

Previous Systematic Reviews

Our comprehensive search identified eight previously published systematic review articles that evaluated the effects of acupuncture for abortive treatment for acute migraine ($n = 1$)[1] and preventive treatment for episodic migraine ($n = 7$).[2–8] Two reviews were published in English[2,3] and the remaining six reviews were published in Chinese. No systematic review on other CM therapies was identified.

Pu *et al.* (2016)[1] systematically reviewed the efficacy and safety of acupuncture as an abortive treatment for acute migraine, compared to sham acupuncture. Five RCTs, published in Chinese ($n = 3$) and English ($n = 2$), were included in this review. The risk of bias tool of the Cochrane method for intervention[9] was applied to assess the methodological quality of included studies. According to meta-analyses, there was no significant difference between acupuncture and sham control for pain visual analogue scales (VAS) at two and four hours after treatment. However, the change score of pain VAS from pre-treatment to post-treatment (at both 2 and 4 hour post-treatment timepoints) of acupuncture groups were superior to that of the sham control. Nevertheless, the small number and low methodological quality of included studies downgraded the certainty of these evidence.

Gao *et al.* (2011) study[4] systematically reviewed the efficacy and safety of real acupuncture versus sham acupuncture as the preventive treatment for episodic migraine. Twelve RCTs were included in the review. The risk of bias of Cochrane tool was applied to assess the methodological quality of the included studies. According to meta-analyses, real acupuncture achieved a higher responder rate after the treatment phase, compared to sham acupuncture; however, this difference was not seen at the end of follow-up. In terms of migraine days, there was no difference between real and sham acupuncture at both post-treatment and post-follow-up timepoints. These results could not be confirmed due to the limitation of 'low' methodological quality of RCTs.

Xian (2013)[5] systematically reviewed the effectiveness and safety of acupuncture as the preventive treatment for episodic migraine. A total of 26 RCTs conducted worldwide, and published in English ($n = 15$) and Chinese ($n = 11$), were included in the review. Three types of comparison were used by the included studies: (1) acupuncture versus no treatment; (2) real acupuncture versus sham acupuncture; and (3) acupuncture versus pharmacotherapy. When acupuncture is compared to no treatment (waiting list), favourable effects of acupuncture were shown at some post-treatment timepoints for one or more outcomes: responder rate, migraine frequency, total migraine days, headache intensity and quality of life (QoL). Compared to sham acupuncture, real acupuncture was superior at some timepoints for responder rate, migraine days, frequency of migraine attack, headache intensity and the Migraine Disability Assessment (MIDAS), but not for the usage of acute medication, duration of an average migraine attack, Pain Disability Index (PDI) and the Short Form (36) Health Survey (SF36). While comparing acupuncture with pharmacotherapy, it was found that acupuncture was more effective for responder rate, frequency of migraine, days of total migraine, headache intensity, PDI, MIDAS and the physical functioning domain of SF36, but not for the rescue medicine consumption and the emotional functioning domain of SF36. However, the superior effects were not consistently shown at all timepoints for all outcome measures. Further research to confirm the effects are required.

Yang *et al.* (2014)[6] systematically reviewed the effectiveness and safety of acupuncture as the preventive treatment for episodic migraine compared to flunarizine. Ten RCTs published in Chinese were included in the review. The methodological quality of included studies was evaluated by the risk of bias of the Cochrane tool. According to meta-analyses, acupuncture had a significant higher responder rate than flunarizine after both treatment and follow-up. In addition, acupuncture could decrease the headache intensity. Few mild AEs were reported in both groups. Due to the limitations of including small number of studies, 'low' methodological quality and inconsistent outcome measures, the evidence provided by this review was not conclusive.

Linde *et al.* (2016)[2] systematically reviewed the effectiveness and safety of acupuncture. Twenty-two RCTs including 4,985 participants met the inclusion criteria of the review. The methodological quality was assessed by using the risk of bias of the Cochrane tool. According to the meta-analyses, when compared to no treatment, acupuncture showed effects in reducing headache frequency and increasing responder rate. When compared to sham acupuncture, real acupuncture achieved greater effects in terms of migraine frequency and responder rate. Using pharmacotherapy as comparison, it was found that acupuncture was superior for the outcome of responder rate for both post-treatment and post-follow-up, as well as for migraine frequency, but this was not maintained until the end of follow-up. It should be noted that, trial participants who received acupuncture were less likely to report AEs or to drop out due to AEs. According to this evidence, authors of the review suggested that adding acupuncture to symptomatic treatment of attacks is beneficial and there is a small effect over sham acupuncture. In addition, acupuncture may be at least similarly effective as the treatment of prophylactic drugs.

Song (2016)[7] systematically reviewed the effectiveness and safety of acupuncture as the preventive treatment for episodic migraine compared to pharmacotherapy. A total of 18 RCTs with 1,470 participants were included in the review. The methodological quality of the included studies was assessed using the risk of bias of the Cochrane tool. According to meta-analyses, acupuncture is superior to pharmacotherapy in increasing responder rate after treatment and at follow-up period. In addition, AEs were less reported in acupuncture groups. However, none of the included studies were published in international journals. The effects of acupuncture need further confirmation by rigorously designed RCTs.

Yang *et al.* (2016)[3] systematically reviewed the efficacy and safety of real acupuncture versus sham acupuncture as the preventive treatment for episodic migraine. Ten RCTs with 997 participants, published in Chinese and English, were included in the review. The methodological quality of the included trials was evaluated by the risk of bias tool. According to the meta-analyses, real acupuncture showed a significant superior effect on the total effective rate, but no significant differences was seen in headache intensity, frequency or duration, accompanying symptoms and usage of medication. No severe AEs related to acupuncture occurred during treatment with either real or sham acupuncture. It seems that real acupuncture is superior to sham acupuncture for migraine.

Chen *et al.* (2018) study[8] systematically reviewed the effectiveness of acupuncture as the preventive treatment for episodic migraine compared to pharmacotherapy. In total, 18 RCTs published in Chinese since 2000 were included in the review. The Jadad scale was used to assess the methodological quality of included studies. Meta-analyses suggested that participants receiving acupuncture had a higher responder rate and fewer AEs than those treated with pharmacotherapy. Due to the limitations of lacking 'high' methodological quality trials, the authors suggested that more rigorously designed RCTs are required to confirm the evidence of acupuncture.

Identification of Clinical Studies

The search of nine English and Chinese language databases identified 10,753 citations, of which 1,348 required full-text retrieval to determine eligibility for inclusion (Fig. 7.1). After assessment against rigorous inclusion criteria, 50 randomised controlled studies evaluating the efficacy and safety of acupuncture for migraine were included in our evaluation. Of all included studies, 39 studies (A1, A3–A40) assessed the effects of acupuncture for preventing episodic migraine, one study (A2) evaluated the effects of acupuncture for both acute migraine management and episodic migraine prevention and another

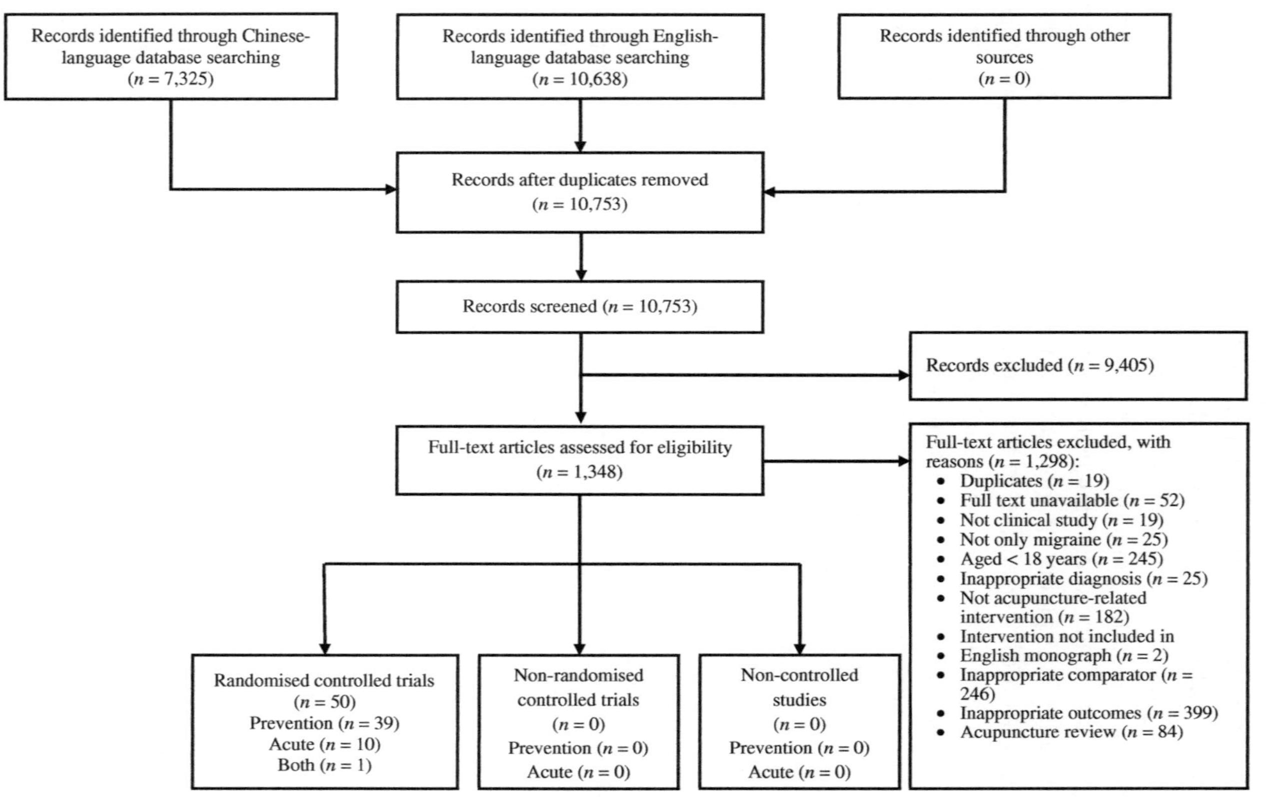

Fig. 7.1. Flowchart of study selection process: Acupuncture

ten studies (A41–A50) evaluated the effects of acupuncture for acute migraine management (Fig. 7.1). The acupuncture therapies used by these studies were body acupuncture (the main type of acupuncture therapy, namely acupuncture thereafter) (46 studies), scalp acupuncture (three studies), ear acupuncture (one study) and heat stimulation on acupuncture points (one study).

In addition, two studies were identified utilising acupuncture-related interventions not commonly practised outside China; the results of these studies are not presented in this chapter.

Acupuncture for Migraine Prevention: Randomised Controlled Trials

In total, 39 RCTs (A1, A3–A40) assessed the effects of acupuncture as the preventive treatment for episodic migraine; one RCT (A2) used acupuncture as both preventive treatment for episodic migraine and abortive treatment for acute migraine. There were no non-randomised controlled trials or non-controlled clinical studies identified meeting our selective criteria. Three of included RCTs (A26, A36, A37) were designed as three-armed studies which contained multiple comparisons; thus the data of these three studies were exacted and analysed in line with the categories of comparisons.

A total of 4,528 participants were included in the 40 RCTs. Among the studies which provided information of participants' gender, there were more females than males (3,410 versus 1,080). The age of all patients included in these studies ranged from 18 years (A5) to 65 years of age (A31, A34, A35), with an average age being 37.36 years.

Of all included RCTs, two studies (A36, A37) compared acupuncture to blank group (no treatment or waiting list), ten studies (A1, A4, A12, A22, A26, A33, A36–A38, A40) compared real acupuncture to sham acupuncture, 17 studies (A3, A7, A10, A11, A14, A17–A19, A21, A23–A27, A32, A34, A35) compared acupuncture to pharmacotherapies and ten RCTs (A5, A8, A9, A13, A15, A20, A28–A31) evaluated the add-on effects of acupuncture to the same pharmacotherapies. One study (A39) compared verum acupuncture plus placebo to sham acupuncture plus real drug and one RCT (A16) evaluated the add-on effect of ear acupuncture to the same pharmacotherapy. The efficacy of acupuncture was analysed and presented below under each category of comparison.

The treatment duration ranged from 28 days (A1–A3, A5, A6, A8–A10, A12–A17, A22, A25, A27, A33, A37, A39) to 180 days (A11), with an average treatment duration being 40.57 days.

The pharmacotherapies for migraine prevention used in these studies as comparators are mainly of three categories: (1) calcium channel blocker ($n = 24$); (2) β-blocker ($n = 4$); (3) antidepressants ($n = 1$); and (4) triptans ($n = 1$). All these pharmacotherapies are recommended by clinical guidelines as the preventive treatment for migraine.[10]

Scalp acupuncture was involved in three RCTs (A8, A15, A21), with two studies (A8, A15) applying only scalp acupuncture, and one study (A21) applying scalp acupuncture together with body acupuncture.

One RCT (A18) recruited participants of one specific syndrome (Liver *yang* uprising 肝阳上亢). Most of the other studies mentioned that modification of acupuncture point selection was allowed according to syndrome differentiation.

All studies reported the names of acupuncture points, except for one study (A26). The frequently used acupuncture points are presented in Table 7.1, of which, the majority is from the Gallbladder and *San jiao* 三焦 (Triple Energizer) meridians. As shown in Table 7.1, acupuncture points located at the head and neck area are more often used than distal points located on limbs.

Risk of Bias Assessment

In total, 22 RCTs (A1, A3, A4, A6, A7, A9–A13, A16, A20, A22, A24–A26, A30, A31, A34–A37) applied appropriate randomisation sequence generation and therefore they were rated as 'low' risk of bias for sequence generation. Five studies (A2, A18, A28, A29, A33) allocated participants based on their sequence of attending; they

Table 7.1. Frequently Reported Acupoints in Randomised Controlled Trials for Migraine Prevention

Most Common Acupuncture Points	Frequency of Use
GB20 *Fengchi* 风池	23
GB8 *Shuaigu* 率谷	21
EX-HN5 *Taiyang* 太阳	16
TE5 *Waiguan* 外关	14
LR3 *Taichong* 太冲	13
LI4 *Hegu* 合谷	13
GV20 *Baihui* 百会	12
GB34 *Yanglingquan* 阳陵泉	12
GB40 *Qiuxu* 丘墟	10
GB41 *Zulinqi* 足临泣	9
ST8 *Touwei* 头维	7
TE20 *Jiaosun* 角孙	7
TE23 *Sizhukong* 丝竹空	6
Ashi points 阿是穴	6
BL60 *Kunlun* 昆仑	5

were assessed as 'high' risk of bias for this item. The remaining 13 studies (A5, A8, A14, A15, A17, A19, A21, A23, A27, A32, A38–A40) were 'unclear' risk of bias for sequence generation since they did not provide sufficient information.

For allocation concealment, 12 studies (A6, A8, A9, A10, A12, A13, A18, A26, A36, A37, A39, A40) were assessed as 'low' risk of bias, because they used opaque envelopes or central randomisation by using a central allocation system; the remaining 28 studies were 'unclear' risk of bias due to lack of information.

In terms of blinding (participants and outcome assessors), only two studies (A6, A39) were assessed as 'low' risk of bias for both items since they applied appropriate sham control, one study (A33) was of 'unclear' risk of bias due to lack of information and the remaining studies were 'high' risk of bias because of inappropriate placebo control.

Table 7.2. Risk of Bias of Randomised Controlled Trials: Acupuncture for Migraine Prevention

Risk of Bias Domain	Low Risk n (%)	Unclear Risk n (%)	High Risk n (%)
Sequence generation	22(55)	13(32.5)	5(12.5)
Allocation concealment	12(30)	28(70)	0(0)
Blinding of participants	2(5)	1(2.5)	37(32.5)
Blinding of personnel	0(0)	0(0)	40(100)
Blinding of outcome assessors	2(5)	1(2.5)	37(32.5)
Incomplete outcome data	35(87.5)	1(2.5)	4(10)
Selective outcome reporting	4(10)	36(90)	0(0)

As for blinding of personnel, all the RCTs were assessed as 'high' risk of bias since the clinical doctors had to be aware of the treatment methods.

In terms of incomplete outcome data, four studies (A6, A8, A9, A14) were judged as 'high' risk of bias because they had high drop-out rate and did not use intention-to-treat (ITT) analysis; one (A33) was judged as 'unclear' risk of bias since there was no information to judge and the remaining were judged as 'low' risk of bias since their low drop-out rate or no drop-out did not affect the outcome results.

For selective reporting, four studies (A26, A36, A37, A39) were judged as 'low' risk of bias because they reported all outcomes as stated in their methods section; the other 36 studies were 'unclear' risk of bias because they did not report publication or registration of their protocol. See Table 7.2 for details.

Outcomes

Outcome measures reported by these studies include monthly migraine frequency, migraine days, migraine duration, pain VAS or numeric rating scale (NRS), responder rate, acute medication usage and QoL. The treatment effects of acupuncture were analysed by pooling the studies of same comparison into meta-analyses. Details of results are shown below under the following categories of comparison:

- Acupuncture versus no treatment or waiting list (*n* = 2);
- Verum acupuncture versus sham acupuncture (*n* = 10);
- Acupuncture versus pharmacotherapy (*n* = 17);
- Acupuncture plus pharmacotherapy versus pharmacotherapy alone (*n* = 9);
- Verum acupuncture plus placebo drug versus sham acupuncture plus real drug (*n* = 1);
- Ear acupuncture plus drug versus drug alone (*n* = 1).

Acupuncture versus No Treatment (Waiting List) (*n* = 2)

Two studies (A36, A37) involving 386 participants compared acupuncture with no treatment (waiting list). Meta-analyses showed that the acupuncture group achieved greater effects than no treatment for migraine days and pain VAS/NRS at the end of treatment. However, data of end of follow-up phase was lacking to prove the long-term benefits of acupuncture to no treatment (see Table 7.3).

Verum Acupuncture versus Sham Acupuncture (*n* = 10)

When comparing verum acupuncture with sham acupuncture, it was found that, at the end of treatment phase, verum acupuncture was

Table 7.3.   Acupuncture versus No Treatment

Outcome	No. of Studies	No. of Participants	Effect Size (RR or MD [95% CI], I²)	Included Studies
Migraine days (monthly), end of treatment	2	386	MD: −1.85 [−2.51, −1.20]*, 27%	A36, A37
Pain VAS/NRS, end of treatment	2	386	MD: −1.59 [−2.18, −1.00]*, 55%	A36, A37

*Statistically significant.

Abbreviations: CI, confidence interval; MD, mean difference; NRS, numeric rating scale; RR, risk ratio; VAS, visual analogue scale.

more effective than sham acupuncture for pain VAS/NRS, but the superiority was not maintained at the end of follow-up phase. For all three domains of Migraine-specific Quality of life Questionnaire (MSQ) scores, verum acupuncture was proved to be more effective than sham acupuncture throughout the treatment and follow-up period. In terms of the migraine frequency, migraine days, responder rate and migraine duration, there is no significant difference between the two groups for both the end of treatment phase and follow-up phase (see Table 7.4).

Table 7.4. Verum Acupuncture versus Sham Acupuncture

Outcome	No. of Studies	No. of Participants	Effect Size (RR or MD [95% CI], I^2)	Included Studies
Migraine frequency (monthly), end of treatment	2	379	MD: −0.67 [−1.85, 0.50], 91%	A22, A36
Migraine frequency (monthly), end of follow-up	2	379	MD: −0.42 [−1.67, 0.84], 92%	A22, A36
Migraine days (monthly), end of treatment	4	474	MD: −1.18 [−2.55, 0.19], 79%	A36–A38, A40
Migraine days (monthly), end of follow-up	4	474	MD: −0.94 [−2.30, 0.43], 76%	A36–A38, A40
Responder rate, end of treatment	2	276	RR: 1.48 [0.58, 3.79], 86%	A36, A40
Responder rate, end of follow-up	3	883	RR: 1.25 [0.82, 1.90], 79%	A26, A36, A40
Migraine duration, end of treatment	2	85	MD: −2.02 [−4.21, 0.18], 0%	A38, A40
Migraine duration, end of follow-up	2	85	MD: −0.66 [−2.62, 1.29], 0%	A38, A40

Table 7.4.   (*Continued*)

Outcome	No. of Studies	No. of Participants	Effect Size (RR or MD [95% CI], I^2)	Included Studies
Pain VAS/NRS, end of treatment	8	813	MD: −0.69 [−1.00, −0.39]*, 54%	A1, A4, A12, A22, A33, A36, A37, A40
Pain VAS/NRS, end of follow-up	5	656	MD: −0.93 [−2.09, 0.24], 95%	A1, A22, A36, A37, A40
MSQ score: Restrictive, end of treatment	7	586	MD: 8.01 [5.83, 10.18]*, 95%	A1, A2, A12, A22, A33, A37, A40
MSQ score: Restrictive, end of follow-up	2	109	MD: 24.80 [19.60, 29.99]*, 49%	A1, A40
MSQ score: Preventive, end of treatment	7	586	MD: 8.37 [6.13, 10.62]*, 93%	A1, A2, A12, A22, A33, A37, A40
MSQ score: Preventive, end of follow-up	2	109	MD: 23.37 [17.76, 28.98]*, 28%	A1, A40
MSQ score: Emotional, end of treatment	7	586	MD: 6.01 [3.73, 8.28]*, 89%	A1, A2, A12, A22, A33, A37, A40
MSQ score: Emotional, end of follow-up	2	109	MD: 21.93 [16.58, 27.28]*, 0%	A1, A40

*Statistically significant.
Abbreviations: CI, confidence interval; MD, mean difference; MSQ, Migraine-specific Quality-of-life Questionnaire; NRS, numeric rating scale; RR, risk ratio; VAS, visual analogue scale.

Acupuncture versus Pharmacotherapy (*n* = 17)

In total 17 studies compared acupuncture with pharmacotherapies recommended by clinical guidelines. According to meta-analyses, at the end of treatment phase, the acupuncture group achieved greater improvement than pharmacotherapies for migraine frequency, migraine

Table 7.5. Acupuncture versus Pharmacotherapy

Outcome	No. of Studies	No. of Participants	Effect Size (RR or MD [95% CI], I^2)	Included Studies
Migraine frequency (monthly), end of treatment	7	708	MD: −1.10 [−1.46, −0.73]*, 88%	A7, A10, A19, A21, A23, A27, A32
Migraine duration, end of treatment	7	709	MD: −10.90 [−18.38, −3.41]*, 99%	A7, A10, A18, A19, A21, A27, A32
Pain VAS/NRS, end of treatment	5	423	MD: −1.32 [−2.18, −0.45]*, 94%	A3, A17, A25, A34, A35
Pain VAS/NRS, end of follow-up	2	179	MD: −1.92 [−3.31, −0.53]*, 93%	A24, A25
MSQ score: Restrictive, end of treatment	2	230	MD: −0.27 [−0.35, −0.19]*, 78%	A11, A14
MSQ score: Preventive, end of treatment	2	230	MD: −0.27 [−0.35, −0.20]*, 56%	A11, A14
MSQ score: Emotional, end of treatment	2	230	MD: −0.28 [−0.35, −0.20]*, 83%	A11, A14

*Statistically significant.
Abbreviations: CI, confidence interval; MD, mean difference; MSQ, Migraine-specific Quality-of-life Questionnaire; NRS, numeric rating scale; VAS, visual analogue scale.

duration and pain VAS/NRS. However, acupuncture was less effective, compared to pharmacotherapy, in terms of MSQ scores. At the end of the follow-up phase, acupuncture was more effective than pharmaco-therapies in reducing pain VAS. There were no data available for meta-analysis to confirm the long-term effect (see Table 7.5)

Acupuncture plus Pharmacotherapy versus Pharmacotherapy Alone (*n* = 10)

When acupuncture was used as an add-on therapy in combination with pharmacotherapy, using the same pharmacotherapy as com-parator, it was found by meta-analyses that adding acupuncture

Table 7.6. Acupuncture plus Pharmacotherapy versus Pharmacotherapy Alone

Outcome	No. of Studies	No. of Participants	Effect Size (MD [95% CI], I^2)	Included Studies
Migraine frequency (monthly), end of treatment	2	122	−2.08 [−3.04, −1.13]*, 72%	A5, A31
Pain VAS/NRS, end of treatment	7	562	−1.18 [−2.38, −0.02]*, 97%	A8, A9, A15, A20, A28, A29, A31
Pain VAS/NRS, end of follow-up	2	148	−2.35 [−2.97, −1.72]*, 0%	A8, A9

*Statistically significant.

Abbreviation: CI, confidence interval; MD, mean difference; NRS, numeric rating scale; VAS, visual analogue scale.

increased the effects for migraine frequency at end-of-treatment phase and pain VAS/NRS at both the end-of-treatment and follow-up phases (see Table 7.6).

Verum Acupuncture plus Placebo Drug versus Sham Acupuncture plus Real Drug (*n* = 1)

Only one RCT (A39) compared the combination of verum acupuncture and placebo drug to the combination of sham acupuncture and flunarizine. The purpose of such a design was to conduct a 'double-dummy' trial to ensure blinding, and that participants of both groups 'could receive effective treatment'. Findings from this study showed that verum acupuncture plus placebo drug was more effective than sham acupuncture plus flunarizine for the outcomes of responder rate at both the end-of-treatment and follow-up periods and for pain VAS at the end of a four-week treatment phase.

Ear Acupuncture plus Drug versus Drug Alone (*n* = 1)

One RCT (A17), involving 160 participants, evaluated the add-on effectiveness of ear acupuncture using flunarizine as a comparator. At the end of the four-week treatment, there was no significant difference between the two groups for pain VAS.

Assessment Using Grading of Recommendations Assessment, Development and Evaluation

Using the Grading of Recommendations Assessment, Development and Evaluation (GRADE) approach, the evidence of most outcomes of acupuncture versus sham was assessed as 'moderate' certainty (see Table 7.7), while the evidence of acupuncture being used as an add-on therapy was assessed as 'very low' to 'low' certainty (see Table 7.8).

Table 7.7.   GRADE: Acupuncture versus Sham for Migraine Prevention

Outcome	Absolute Effect		Relative Effect (95% CI) No. of Participants (Studies)	Certainty of the Evidence (GRADE)
	Acupuncture	Sham Acupuncture		
Migraine frequency (monthly), end of treatment	**1.63** MD: 0.67 lower (95% CI: 1.85 lower to 0.5 higher)	2.3	**MD −0.67** (−1.85, 0.5) 379 (2 RCTs)	⊕⊕◯◯ LOW[1,2]
Migraine frequency (monthly), end of follow-up	**1.79** MD: 0.42 lower (95% CI: 1.67 lower to 0.84 higher)	2.21	**MD −0.42** (−1.67, 0.84) 379 (2 RCTs)	⊕⊕◯◯ LOW[1,2]
Migraine days (monthly), end of treatment	**4.72** MD: 1.18 lower (95% CI: 2.55 lower to 0.19 higher)	5.9	**MD −1.18** (−2.55, 0.19) 474 (4 RCTs)	⊕⊕⊕◯ MODERATE[1]
Migraine days (monthly), end of follow-up	**4.49** MD: 0.94 lower (95% CI: 2.3 lower to 0.43 higher)	5.43	**MD −0.94** (−2.3, +0.43) 474 (4 RCTs)	⊕⊕⊕◯ MODERATE[1]
Responder rate, end of treatment	**71** per 100 Difference: 23 more per 100 patients (95% CI: 20 fewer to 100 more per 100 patients)	48 per 100	**RR 1.48** (0.58, 3.79) 276 (2 RCTs)	⊕⊕◯◯ LOW[1,2]

Table 7.7. (*Continued*)

Outcome	Absolute Effect		Relative Effect (95% CI) No. of Participants (Studies)	Certainty of the Evidence (GRADE)
	Acupuncture	Sham Acupuncture		
Responder rate, end of follow-up	**50** per 100	**40** per 100	**RR 1.25** (0.82, 1.9)	⊕⊕⊕○ MODERATE[1]
	Difference: 10 more per 100 patients (95% CI: 7 fewer to 36 more per 100 patients)		883 (3 RCTs)	
Pain VAS/NRS, end of treatment	**3.58** MD: 0.69 lower (95% CI: 1 lower to 0.39 lower)	**4.27**	**MD −0.69** (−1, −0.39) 813 (8 RCTs)	⊕⊕⊕⊕ HIGH
Pain VAS/NRS, end of follow-up	**2.91** MD: 0.93 lower (95% CI: 2.09 lower to 0.24 higher)	**3.84**	**MD −0.93** (−2.09, 0.24) 656 (5 RCTs)	⊕⊕⊕○ MODERATE[1]
MSQ score: Restrictive, end of treatment	**74.05** MD: 8.01 higher (95% CI: 5.83 higher to 10.18 higher)	**66.04**	**MD 8.01** (5.83, 10.18) 586 (7 RCTs)	⊕⊕⊕○ MODERATE[1]
MSQ score: Restrictive, end of follow-up	**82.6** MD: 24.8 higher (95% CI: 19.6 higher to 29.99 higher)	**57.8**	**MD 24.8** (19.6, 29.99) 109 (2 RCTs)	⊕⊕⊕○ MODERATE[2]
MSQ score: Preventive, end of treatment	**82.85** MD: 8.37 higher (95% CI: 6.13 higher to 10.62 higher)	**74.48**	**MD 8.37** (6.13, 10.62) 586 (7 RCTs)	⊕⊕⊕○ MODERATE[1]
MSQ score: Preventive, end of follow-up	**88.62** MD: 23.37 higher (95% CI: 17.76 higher to 28.98 higher)	**65.25**	**MD 23.37** (17.76, 28.98) 109 (2 RCTs)	⊕⊕⊕○ MODERATE[2]

(*Continued*)

Table 7.7.   (*Continued*)

Outcome	Absolute Effect		Relative Effect (95% CI) No. of Participants (Studies)	Certainty of the Evidence (GRADE)
	Acupuncture	Sham Acupuncture		
MSQ score: Emotional and Functional, end of treatment	**80.9** MD: 6.01 higher (95% CI: 3.73 higher to 8.28 higher)	**74.89**	**MD 6.01** (3.73, 8.28) 586 (7 RCTs)	⊕⊕⊕◯ MODERATE[1]
MSQ score: Emotional and Functional, end of follow-up	**88.22** MD: 21.93 higher (95% CI: 16.58 higher to 27.28 higher)	**66.29**	**MD 21.93** (16.58, 27.28) 109 (2 RCTs)	⊕⊕⊕◯ MODERATE[2]

The risk in the intervention group (and its 95% confidence interval) is based on the assumed risk in the comparison group and the relative effect of the intervention (and its 95% CI).
Abbreviations: CI, confidence interval; MD, mean difference; MSQ, Migraine-specific Quality-of-life Questionnaire; NRS, numeric rating scale; RCT(s), randomised controlled trial(s); RR, risk ratio; VAS, visual analogue scale.

Notes

[1]High heterogeneity may limit the certainty of results.
[2]Small sample size may limit the certainty of results.

Study references
Migraine frequency (monthly), end of treatment: A22, A36.
Frequency of migraine (monthly), end of follow-up: A22, A36.
Migraine days (monthly), end of treatment: A36–A38, A40.
Migraine days (monthly), end of follow-up: A36–A38, A40.
Responder rate, end of treatment: A36, A40.
Responder rate, end of follow-up: A26, A36, A40.
Pain VAS/NRS, end of treatment: A1, A4, A12, A22, A33, A36, A37, A40.
Pain VAS/NRS, end of follow-up: A1, A22, A36, A37, A40.
MSQ score: Restrictive, end of treatment: A1, A2, A12, A22, A33, A37, A40.
MSQ score: Restrictive: end of follow-up: A1, A40.
MSQ score: Preventive, end of treatment: A1, A2, A12, A22, A33, A37, A40.
MSQ score: Preventive: end of follow-up: A1, A40.
MSQ score: Emotional and Functional, end of treatment: A1, A2, A12, A22, A33, A37, A40.
MSQ score: Emotional and Functional, end of follow-up: A1, A40.

Table 7.8. GRADE: Acupuncture plus Pharmacotherapy versus Pharmacotherapy Alone for Migraine Prevention

Outcome	Absolute Effect		Relative Effect (95% CI) No. of Participants (Studies)	Certainty of the Evidence (GRADE)
	Acupuncture plus Pharmacotherapy	**Pharmacotherapy**		
Migraine frequency (monthly), end of treatment	**1.8** MD: 2.08 lower (95% CI: 3.04 to 1.13 lower)	**3.88**	**MD −2.08** (−3.04, −1.13) 122 (2 RCTs)	⊕○○○ VERY LOW[1,2,3]
Migraine days (monthly), end of treatment	**1.3** MD: 2.56 lower (95% CI: 2.93 to 2.18 lower)	**3.86**	**MD −2.56** (−2.93, −2.18) 68 (1 RCT)	⊕⊕○○ LOW[1,3]
Pain VAS/NRS, end of treatment	**3.16** MD: 1.18 lower (95% CI: 2.38 lower to 0.02 lower)	**4.34**	**MD −1.18** (−2.38, −0.02) 562 (7 RCTs)	⊕⊕○○ LOW[1,2]
Pain VAS/NRS, end of follow-up	**3.8** MD: 2.35 lower (95% CI: 2.97 to 1.72 lower)	**6.15**	**RR −2.35** (−2.97, −1.72) 148 (2 RCTs)	⊕⊕○○ LOW[1,3]
MIDAS, end of treatment	**2.1** MD: 6.9 lower (95% CI: 8.06 to 5.74 lower)	**9**	**MD −6.9** (−8.06, −5.74) 66 (1 RCT)	⊕⊕○○ LOW[1,3]
MIDAS, end of follow-up	**2.2** MD: 6.7 lower (95% CI: 7.81 to 5.59 lower)	**8.9**	**MD −6.7** (−7.81, −5.59) 66 (1 RCT)	⊕⊕○○ LOW[1,3]

The risk in the intervention group (and its 95% confidence interval) is based on the assumed risk in the comparison group and the relative effect of the intervention (and its 95% CI).

Abbreviations: CI, confidence interval; MD, mean difference; MIDAS, Migraine Disability Assessment; NRS, numeric rating scale; RCT(s), randomised controlled trial(s); VAS, visual analogue scale.

Notes

[1]High risk of bias in blinding may influence the result.
[2]High heterogeneity may limit the certainty of results.
[3]Small sample size may limit the certainty of results.

Study references
Migraine frequency (monthly), end of treatment: A5, A31.
Migraine days (monthly), end of treatment: A31.
Pain VAS/NRS, end of treatment: A8, A9, A15, A20, A28, A29, A31.
Pain VAS/NRS, end of follow-up: A8, A9.
MIDAS, end of treatment: A30.
MIDAS, end of follow-up: A30.

Frequently Reported Acupuncture Points in Meta-analyses Showing Favourable Effect

To show which acupuncture points may have contributed to the meta-analyses with favourable effects towards acupuncture, the studies included in those meta-analyses were pooled for acupuncture point frequency analyses. Since there were multiple meta-analyses of different comparisons and outcomes, the acupuncture point analyses were based on outcomes in the same category regardless of the comparisons and the timepoint of outcome assessment. Results are shown in Table 7.9.

Table 7.9. Frequently Reported Acupuncture Points in Meta-analyses Showing Favourable Effect for Migraine Prevention

Outcome Measure	No. of Meta-analyses	No. of Studies	Acupuncture Points	Frequency of Use
Migraine frequency, migraine duration, migraine days (monthly)	4	13	GB20 *Fengchi* 风池	11
			GB8 *Shuaigu* 率谷	9
			TE5 *Waiguan* 外关	7
			GB41 *Zulinqi* 足临泣	7
			LI4 *Hegu* 合谷	7
			TE23 *Sizhukong* 丝竹空	6
			LR3 *Taichong* 太冲	6
			GB34 *Yanglingquan* 阳陵泉	6
			EX-HN5 *Taiyang* 太阳	6
			GB40 *Qiuxu* 丘墟	5
Migraine pain, VAS/NRS	7	28	GB20 *Fengchi* 风池	15
			GB8 *Shuaigu* 率谷	13
			EX-HN5 *Taiyang* 太阳	12
			LR3 *Taichong* 太冲	10
			LI4 *Hegu* 合谷	10
			TE5 *Waiguan* 外关	8
			GB40 *Qiuxu* 丘墟	7
			GV20 *Baihui* 百会	7
			GB34 *Yanglingquan* 阳陵泉	6

Table 7.9. (*Continued*)

Outcome Measure	No. of Meta-analyses	No. of Studies	Acupuncture Points	Frequency of Use
QoL: MSQ	6	8	GB40 *Qiuxu* 丘墟	5
			GB34 *Yanglingquan* 阳陵泉	5
			TE5 *Waiguan* 外关	4
			TE20 *Jiaosun* 角孙	4

Abbreviations: MSQ, Migraine-specific Quality-of-life Questionnaire; NRS, numeric rating scale; QoL, quality of life; VAS, visual analogue scale.

There were 13 RCTs included in four meta-analyses which achieved significant favourable effects of acupuncture for migraine frequency, duration and migraine days. The most frequently used points of these studies were GB20 *Fengchi* 风池, GB8 *Shuaigu* 率谷, TE5 *Waiguan* 外关, GB41 *Zulinqi* 足临泣, TE23 *Sizhukong* 丝竹空, LI4 *Hegu* 合谷, LR3 *Taichong* 太冲, GB34 *Yanglingquan* 阳陵泉, GB40 *Qiuxu* 丘墟 and EX-HN5 *Taiyang* 太阳.

When pooling 28 studies which contributed to the positive meta-analysis of pain VAS/NRS, the most frequently used points were GB20 *Fengchi* 风池, GB8 *Shuaigu* 率谷, EX-HN5 *Taiyang* 太阳, LR3 *Taichong* 太冲, LI4 *Hegu* 合谷, TE5 *Waiguan* 外关, GB40 *Qiuxu* 丘墟, GV20 *Baihui* 百会 and GB34 *Yanglingquan* 阳陵泉. In terms of QoL assessment (MSQ), eight RCTs were included in six meta-analyses showing favourable effects of acupuncture. The most frequent points used by these studies were GB40 *Qiuxu* 丘墟, GB34 *Yanglingquan* 阳陵泉, TE5 *Waiguan* 外关 and TE20 *Jiaosun* 角孙.

According to the frequency analyses, it was found that most of the preferred acupuncture points used by RCTs were located in the Gallbladder and *San jiao* 三焦 (Triple Energizer) meridians, which is the same as that of all included RCTs (see Table 7.1). Tracing back to meridian theory in classical and modern literature, unilateral headache is believed to be a disorder of the *Shao yang* 少阳 meridians. This theory has been guiding our clinical practice for thousands of years.

Acupuncture for Acute Migraine Management

Ten RCTs (A41–A50) investigated the effectiveness of acupuncture as abortive treatment for acute migraine. One RCT (A2) evaluated the effects of acupuncture for both acute migraine management and episodic migraine prevention; the data of acupuncture used as abortive treatment is also pooled for analysis. A total of 1,244 participants were included in these 11 studies. According to the gender information collected from the RCTs, the number of females was more than twice that of males (677 versus 286, respectively). The age of all participants involved in the studies ranged from 18 years (A44, A45) to 75 years (A45), with an average age being 35.4 years old.

Of all included RCTs, four studies (A2, A41, A42, A50) compared verum acupuncture to sham acupuncture, six studies (A43–A47, A49) compared acupuncture to pharmacotherapy and one study (A48) evaluated the add-on effect of heat stimulation on acupuncture points to pharmacotherapy. The efficacy of acupuncture was analysed and presented below under each category of comparison.

The treatment duration ranged from 20 minutes (A48) to one hour (A43, A45), with an average treatment duration being 34.5 minutes. The pharmacotherapies for migraine abortive treatment used in these studies as comparators are mainly of two categories: (1) migraine-specific painkillers for migraine, such as triptans ($n = 3$) and (2) non-specific pain medicine such ergotamine or caffeine/ergotamine.

Only two studies (A44, A47) recruited participants of migraine with a specific CM syndrome, Liver *yang* uprising 肝阳上亢, and tailored their treatments targeting this syndrome. The most frequently used acupuncture points were analysed (see Table 7.10).

Risk of Bias

Seven RCTs (A41, A42, A44, A45, A47, A48, A50) applied appropriate randomised sequence generation and therefore they were rated as 'low' risk of bias for sequence generation. The remaining four studies (A2, A43, A46, A49) were rated as 'unclear' risk of bias for this since they did not provide sufficient information. For allocation

Table 7.10. Frequently Reported Acupuncture Points in Randomised Controlled Trials for Acute Migraine Management

Most Common Acupuncture Points	Frequency of Use
GB8 *Shuaigu* 率谷	6
GB20 *Fengchi* 风池	6
TE5 *Waiguan* 外关	5
GB34 *Yanglingquan* 阳陵泉	5
EX-HN5 *Taiyang* 太阳	4
GB40 *Qiuxu* 丘墟	3
TE20 *Jiaosun* 角孙	3

concealment, four studies (A41, A42, A44, A50) were 'low' risk of bias because they used opaque envelopes or central randomisation by using a phone messaging system. The remaining seven studies were 'unclear' risk of bias due to lack of information.

In terms of blinding (participants and outcome assessors), only three studies (A2, A41, A42) were assessed as 'low' risk of bias for both items since they applied appropriate sham controls, and the remaining studies were 'high' risk of bias; one (A50) for inappropriate sham control and seven for easily distinguished comparisons.

As for blinding of personnel, all the RCTs were assessed as 'high' risk of bias since the clinical doctors had to be aware of the treating methods. In terms of the 'incomplete outcome data', all studies were judged as 'low' risk of bias since their low drop-out rate or no drop-out did not affect the outcome results.

For selective reporting, only one study (A50) was judged as 'low' risk of bias because it reported all outcomes as stated in their methods section. The remaining studies were 'unclear' risk of bias because they did not report publication or registration of their protocol. See Table 7.11 for details.

Outcomes

Outcome measures reported by these studies include pain VAS/NRS and responder rate. The treatment effects of acupuncture were

Table 7.11. Risk of Bias of Randomised Controlled Trials: Acupuncture for Migraine Acute Management

Risk of Bias Domain	Low Risk *n* (%)	Unclear Risk *n* (%)	High Risk *n* (%)
Sequence generation	7(63.6)	4(36.4)	0(0)
Allocation concealment	4(36.4)	7(63.6)	0(0)
Blinding of participants	3(27.3)	0(0)	8(72.7)
Blinding of personnel	0(0)	0(0)	11(100)
Blinding of outcome assessors	3(27.3)	0(0)	8(72.7)
Incomplete outcome data	11(100)	0(0)	0(0)
Selective outcome reporting	1(9.1)	10(90.9)	0(0)

analysed by pooling the studies of same comparison into meta-analyses. Details of results are shown below under the following categories of comparison:

- Verum acupuncture versus sham acupuncture ($n = 4$);
- Acupuncture versus pharmacotherapy ($n = 6$);
- Heating acupoints plus pharmacotherapy versus pharmacotherapy alone ($n = 1$).

Verum Acupuncture versus Sham Acupuncture ($n = 4$)

Four studies compared verum acupuncture with sham acupuncture. Meta-analyses showed that the verum acupuncture group achieved a greater responder rate than the sham acupuncture group; for pain VAS/NRS there was no significant difference (see Table 7.12).

Acupuncture versus Pharmacotherapy ($n = 6$)

Six studies compared acupuncture with pharmacotherapy. Five studies reported data on pain VAS. Meta-analysis showed that acupuncture achieved a better effect in reducing pain VAS. Three studies reported responder rate according to the meta-analysis result; there was no significant difference between the two treatment methods (see Table 7.13).

Table 7.12. Verum Acupuncture versus Sham Acupuncture

Outcome	No. of Studies	No. of Participants	Effect Size (RR or MD [95% CI], I^2)	Included Studies
Responder rate, end of treatment	2	169	RR: 2.27 [1.02, 5.05]*, 53%	A41, A50
Pain VAS/NRS, end of treatment	3	230	MD: −0.54 [−1.13, 0.05], 66%	A2, A41, A42

*Statistically significant.
Abbreviations: CI, confidence interval; MD, mean difference; NRS, numeric rating scale; RR, risk ratio; VAS, visual analogue scale.

Table 7.13. Acupuncture versus Pharmacotherapy

Outcomes	No. of Studies	No. of Participants	Effect Size (RR or MD [95% CI], I^2)	Included Studies
Responder rate, end of treatment	3	357	RR: 1.05 [0.92, 1.21], 66%	A43, A46, A47
Pain VAS/NRS, end of treatment	5	522	MD: −0.73 [−1.23, −0.23]*, 95%	A43–A46, A49

*Statistically significant.
Abbreviations: CI, confidence interval; MD, mean difference; NRS, numeric rating scale; RR, risk ratio; VAS, visual analogue scale.

Heat Stimulation plus Pharmacotherapy versus Pharmacotherapy Alone (*n* = 1)

Only one study (A48) evaluated the add-on effect of applying heat stimulation on acupuncture points when they were used in combination with pharmacotherapy (sumatriptan). A total of 120 participants were involved in the study. Pain VAS was reported in the study, adding heat stimulation to sumatriptan was not beneficial for pain relief.

Assessment Using Grading of Recommendations Assessment, Development and Evaluation

Using the GRADE approach, the meta-analyses results of acupuncture were assessed as 'moderate' or 'low' certainty (see Table 7.14).

Table 7.14. GRADE: Acupuncture versus Sham Acupuncture for Acute Migraine

Outcome	Absolute Effect		Relative Effect (95% CI) No. of Participants (Studies)	Certainty of the Evidence (GRADE)
	Acupuncture	Sham Acupuncture		
Responder rate, end of treatment	**43** per 100	**19** per 100	**RR 2.27** (1.02, 5.05)	⊕⊕⊕○ MODERATE[1]
	Difference: 24 more per 100 patients (95% CI: 0 to 77 more per 100 patients)		169 (2 RCTs)	
Pain VAS/NRS, end of treatment	**2.74** MD: 0.54 lower (95% CI: 1.13 lower to 0.05 higher)	**3.28**	**MD −0.54** (−1.13, 0.05) 230 (3 RCTs)	⊕⊕○○ LOW[1,2]

The risk in the intervention group (and its 95% confidence interval) is based on the assumed risk in the comparison group and the relative effect of the intervention (and its 95% CI). Abbreviations: CI, confidence interval; MD, mean difference; NRS, numeric rating scale; RCT(s), randomised controlled trial(s); RR, risk ratio; VAS, visual analogue scale.

Notes:

[1]Small sample size limited the certainty of results.
[2]High heterogeneity may limit the certainty of results.

Study references:

Responder rate, end of treatment: A41, A50.
Pain VAS/NRS, end of treatment: A2, A41, A42.

Frequently Reported Acupuncture Points in Meta-analyses Showing Favourable Effect

To summarise which acupuncture points contributed to the meta-analyses with favourable effects towards acupuncture therapies, the studies included in those meta-analyses were pooled for point frequency analyses (see Table 7.15). Overall, seven RCTs were included in two meta-analyses showing favourable effects of acupuncture. The most frequent acupuncture points used by these studies were GB40 *Qiuxu* 丘墟, TE5 *Waiguan* 外关, GB8 *Shuaigu* 率谷, TE20 *Jiaosun* 角孙, GB34 *Yanglingquan* 阳陵泉 and GB20 *Fengchi* 风池.

Table 7.15. Frequently Reported Acupuncture Points in Meta-analyses Showing Favourable Effect for Acute Migraine Management

No. of Meta-analyses	No. of Studies	Acupuncture Points	Frequency of Use
2	7	GB40 *Qiuxu* 丘墟	3
		TE5 *Waiguan* 外关	3
		GB8 *Shuaigu* 率谷	3
		TE20 *Jiaosun* 角孙	3
		GB34 *Yanglingquan* 阳陵泉	3
		GB20 *Fengchi* 风池	3

Just like the analysis of overall acupuncture points frequency and the points in meta-analyses showing favourable effect for migraine prevention (Table 7.9), most of these acupuncture points are from *Shao yang* 少阳 meridians, half are local points and another half are distal points.

Safety of Acupuncture

Among all RCTs, 30 did not mention any information of AEs and 20 reported AEs information. The amount of mild or moderate AEs that occurred in the acupuncture group was less than those in the control group (181 versus 240, respectively). There were nine serious AEs, but they were assessed as not related to acupuncture treatments. More details are listed below in line with the different types of comparison:

- Real acupuncture versus sham acupuncture: The AEs that occurred in both groups were all caused by the needling procedure, such as pain or bleeding of the needling area;
- Acupuncture versus pharmacotherapy: The AEs that occurred in the acupuncture group were pain or bleeding of the needling area, while AE that occurred in the pharmacotherapy group was mainly

drowsiness, which was the commonly reported side effect of the pharmacotherapy;

- Acupuncture add-on to pharmacotherapy: The AEs reported by the combination group were less than those reported by the pharmacotherapy group.

Evidence for Acupuncture Therapy Commonly Used in Clinical Practice

The common practice of acupuncture and other therapy for migraine recommended by clinical guidelines and textbooks are summarised in Chapter 2. Acupuncture was recommended to be applied on local *Ashi* points 阿是穴 or points from *Shao yang* 少阳 meridians as the treatment for acute migraine; electroacupuncture could also be considered. For migraine prevention, acupuncture (or with electroacupuncture) could be applied according to CM syndrome differentiation, in addition to being applied on local *Ashi* points 阿是穴 or points from *Shao yang* 少阳 meridians. Scalp acupuncture is usually used for the acute stage. Ear acupuncture/ acupressure, moxibustion and *tuina* 推拿 therapy can also be considered in clinical practice.

Our comprehensive evaluation found that the majority of clinical studies were of acupuncture, for both acute migraine and migraine prevention. There was only one RCT that evaluated ear acupuncture therapy for migraine prevention and one RCT that evaluated heat stimulation, which is similar to moxibustion therapy, for acute migraine management. Evidence of other therapies recommended in Chapter 2 is lacking.

According to the evidence of clinical studies included in our evaluation, when acupuncture was used for migraine prevention, it was more effective than no treatment (waiting list) for migraine days and pain VAS/NRS at the end-of-treatment phase; it was also more effective than sham acupuncture for pain VAS/NRS at the end-of-treatment phase and beneficial for patients' QoL at both the end-of-treatment and follow-up phases. When compared to pharmacotherapy, acupuncture was more effective for migraine frequency and duration, as well as pain VAS/NRS; however, it was inferior to pharmacotherapy for patients' QoL. Acupuncture was also effective when it was used as an add-on therapy to pharmacotherapy in terms of reducing migraine frequency and pain VAS/NRS.

In these clinical studies, most of the points used were selected from *Shao yang* 少阳 meridians (including the Gallbladder and *San jiao* 三焦 [Triple Energizer] meridians). This is consistent with what was introduced in Chapter 2. Furthermore, acupuncture was also evaluated by clinical studies when it was used for managing acute migraine. Our analyses found that acupuncture was more effective than pharmacotherapy for reducing pain and more effective than sham acupuncture in terms of responder rate. The points used by these studies were similar to those used for prevention acupuncture.

Summary of Acupuncture and Other Therapies Clinical Evidence

Acupuncture therapies and other CM therapies, such as *tuina* 推拿 therapy and moxibustion, are recommended in clinical guidelines for the management of migraine. Through a comprehensive search and rigorous selection process, certain evidence was found supporting the use of acupuncture therapies. However, there is a lack of rigorous evidence to support the use of other CM therapies. The evaluation of the clinical study evidence found support for the use of acupuncture to manage migraine for both the acute stage and prevention. Previously published systematic reviews suggested that acupuncture was more effective than sham acupuncture for acute migraine and more effective than sham or pharmacotherapy for migraine prevention. In addition, acupuncture was an effective add-on therapy for the management of migraine prevention. However, the lack of high-quality trials was the main common issue of previous systematic reviews which prevented the review authors from making definite conclusions.

Based on our evaluation of clinical studies which met our inclusion criteria, there was evidence supporting the use of acupuncture for both acute migraine and migraine prevention in order to reduce pain, monthly migraine frequency and migraine duration, as well as to improve migraine sufferers' QoL. However, most of the included studies did not include a follow-up phase to confirm whether acupuncture has any long-term effects.

Acupuncture points selected are mainly the points from *Shao yang* 少阳 meridians (including the Gallbladder and *San jiao* 三焦 [Triple Energizer] meridians), especially local points such as GB20 *Fengchi* 风池 and GB8 *Shuaigu* 率谷. The average duration of acupuncture treatment was around 40 days to prevent migraine attacks and around 30 minutes for treating acute migraine.

Using the GRADE approach, when comparing acupuncture with sham control, the evidence of most outcomes was assessed as 'moderate' certainty; while when acupuncture was used as an add-on therapy, the evidence was assessed as 'low or 'very low' certainty. This reflected the fact that most of the trials designed as acupuncture versus sham control were of higher quality.

On the other hand, acupuncture is safe in the management of migraine. The commonly seen AEs caused by acupuncture were pain and bleeding in the local area, or dizziness after needling. These AEs could be avoided by improving practitioners' skills. By adding acupuncture to pharmacotherapy, the commonly seen AEs of pharmacotherapy seemed reduced. Therefore, acupuncture can be considered as a safe intervention for migraine, especially for the migraine patients who are suffering severe symptoms of nausea and vomiting and having difficulties taking medications. Furthermore, there were insufficient data of other acupuncture-related therapies used as migraine management.

It was worth noting that, in previous clinical research, around one third of the RCTs compared acupuncture to sham acupuncture, although there were a few different methods of the sham design. One RCT made the effort of designing the trial as a 'double-blinding, double-dummy' one, although this approach has not been widely accepted. It has been acknowledged that an ideal design of placebo acupuncture to ensure double-blinding is challenging.[11,12] The 'double-blinding, double-dummy' design using verum acupuncture plus placebo drug compared to sham acupuncture plus real drug is somehow problematic considering the placebo drug and sham acupuncture may produce therapeutic effects in different degrees.

References

1. 蒲圣雄, 谭戈, 王达岩, *et al.* (2016) 针刺对偏头痛急性发作期止痛疗效 meta 分析. 重庆医学 **45(10):** 1353–1356.

2. Linde K, Allais G, Brinkhaus B, *et al.* (2016) Acupuncture for the prevention of episodic migraine. *Cochrane Database Syst Rev* **(6):** CD001218.

3. Yang Y, Que Q, Ye X, Zheng G. (2016) Verum versus sham manual acupuncture for migraine: A systematic review of randomised controlled trials. *Acupunct Med* **34(2):** 76–83.

4. 高小梅, 王柏松, 宋艳艳, *et al.* (2011) 针刺治疗偏头痛的系统评价和 meta 分析. 中国临床药理学与治疗学 **16(05):** 530–537.

5. 仙晋. (2013) 针刺预防性治疗偏头痛的系统评价与选穴配伍规律的研究 (Thesis). 山东中医药大学.

6. 杨佳, 沈燕, 王舒. (2014) 针刺与氟桂利嗪对偏头痛疗效的系统评价. 世界科学技术: 中医药现代化 **7:** 1608–1613.

7. 宋倩. (2016) 针刺与西药比较预防性治疗偏头痛的 meta 分析. 辽宁中医杂志 **43(4):** 821–826.

8. 陈乐, 何晓婷, 徐海燕, *et al.* (2018) 针灸治疗偏头痛随机对照临床研究文献的 meta 分析. 湖南中医杂志 **34(2):** 125–129.

9. Higgins J, Green S, eds. (2011) Cochrane Handbook for Systematic Reviews of Interventions Version 5.1.0. The Cochrane Collaboration. Available from: http://www.cochrane-handbook.org.

10. 中华医学会疼痛学分会头面痛学组. (2016) 中国偏头痛防治指南. 中国疼痛医学杂志 **22(10):** 721–727.

11. Zhang CS, Tan HY, Zhang GS, *et al.* (2015) Placebo devices as effective control methods in acupuncture clinical trials: A systematic review. *PLoS One* **10(11):** e0140825.

12. Zhang GS, Zhang CS, Tan HY, *et al.* (2018) Systematic review of acupuncture placebo devices with a focus on the credibility of blinding of healthy participants and/or acupuncturists. *Acupunct Med* **36(4):** 204–214.

References to Included Studies

A1   陈慧敏. (2009) 针刺少阳经特定穴治疗偏头痛的临床研究 (Thesis). 湖南中医药大学.

A2   常小荣, 陈选, 严洁, *et al.* (2013) 针刺少阳经特定穴对偏头痛患者远期 VAS 计分和头痛强度及 MSQ 评分的临床观察. 中华中医药杂志 **28(8):** 2414–2416.

A3   屈箫箫, 沈燕. (2015) 针刺和盐酸氟桂利嗪预防性治疗偏头痛疗效对比. 陕西中医 **36(6):** 723–724.

A4   王军, 徐欣, 陈三三, 刘然. (2016) 针刺腧穴痛觉敏感点治疗偏头痛的临床观察. 第二十二届全国针灸临床学术研讨会暨第二届全国针灸学术流派交流研讨会暨河南省针灸学会针灸临床分会 2016 年年会暨河南省针灸临床应用及特色技术学术交流会会议. 中国河南洛阳.

A5   王俊. (2010) 针刺少阳经经穴联合氟桂利嗪治疗偏头痛的临床观察. 湖北中医杂志 **32(4):** 68–69.

A6   王麟鹏. (2009) 针刺治疗偏头痛临床疗效的讨论. 2009 年全国针灸临床学术研讨会暨北京地区针灸名家学术推广会, 北京.

A7   谢菊英, 贺莉萍, 李志宏, 唐伟. (2009) 针刺足少阳经经穴为主治疗偏头痛 31 例临床观察. 中医药导报 **15(04):** 60–61.

A8   杨丽. (2010) 头针配合西药与单纯西药治疗无先兆偏头痛的远期疗效的对照研究 (Thesis). 成都中医药大学.

A9   杨旭光. (2006) 电针 '四关' 穴治疗无先兆偏头痛的近期疗效和远期疗效的临床观察 (Thesis). 成都中医药大学.

A10   钟广伟, 李炜, 罗艳红, *et al.* (2009) 针刺肝胆经穴治疗偏头痛: 多中心随机对照研究. 中国针灸 **29(04):** 259–263.

A11   Allais G, De Lorenzo C, Quirico PE, *et al.* (2002) Acupuncture in the prophylactic treatment of migraine without aura: A comparison with flunarizine. *Headache* **42(9):** 855–861.

A12   蔡涛键. (2016) 平衡针灸针刺无先兆偏头痛患者头痛穴的临床观察 (Thesis). 广州中医药大学.

A13   曾盛锦. (2009) 针刺调神法治疗无先兆偏头痛的临床疗效观察 (Thesis). 成都中医药大学.

A14   戴睛, 江彬, 杨柳, *et al.* (2017) 骨边刺法治疗偏头痛 35 例疗效观察. 浙江中医杂志 **52(9):** 687–688.

A15   段勇明. (2014) 针灸结合西药治疗偏头痛疗效分析. 中国医药科学 **4(16):** 78–79, 112.

(Continued)

A16 侯宝山, 李国宝. (2016) 耳穴压豆法联合盐酸氟桂利嗪胶囊治疗偏头痛. 长春中医药大学学报 **32(5):** 970–972.

A17 李道丕, 姬锋养, 刘鹏, *et al.* (2011) 针刺结合磁珠压耳治疗偏头痛临床观察. 针灸临床杂志 **27(06):** 25–26.

A18 李甘. (2013) 电针预防性治疗偏头痛的临床观察 (Thesis). 湖北中医药大学.

A19 李志宏. (2009) 针刺手少阳经经穴为主治疗偏头痛 32 例临床观察. 湖南中医杂志 **25(2):** 11–12.

A20 林仕彬. (2013) 针刺颈部夹脊穴对偏头痛的疗效观察. 中国伤残医学 **21(8):** 222–223.

A21 刘克英, 刘秀梅, 马成福, *et al.* (2001) 针刺与药物治疗偏头痛临床疗效对比研究. 中国针灸 **21(9):** 515–517.

A22 刘艳琴. (2015) 循经取穴治疗偏头痛的临床持续效应再评价 (Thesis). 成都中医药大学.

A23 倪承浩. (2002) 开 '四关' 治疗无先兆性偏头痛 32 例. 上海中医药大学学报 **16(4):** 24–25.

A24 沈文, 谷婕, 李芳, *et al.* (2017) 水突穴体表电刺激联合指趾端刺治疗偏头痛临床效果随机对照研究. 针灸临床杂志 **33(10):** 34–37.

A25 舒伟, 彭天忠, 黄学娣, *et al.* (2017) 间歇式柔肝调神针刺法预防性治疗偏头痛疗效观察. 上海针灸杂志 **A36(6):** 727–730.

A26 Diener HC, Kronfeld K, Boewing G, *et al.* (2006) Efficacy of acupuncture for the prophylaxis of migraine: A multicentre randomised controlled clinical trial. *Lancet Neurol* **5(4):** 310–316.

A27 田菁. (2006) 头部透穴疗法治疗偏头痛 30 例疗效观察. 实用中医内科杂志 **20(6).**

A28 王志平. (2017) 尼莫地平片联合针刺治疗偏头痛的疗效及安全性观察. 心理医生 **23(16):** 22–23.

A29 吴红晓. (2015) 针灸治疗偏头痛疗效观察. 医药前沿 5(36): 361–362.

A30 Facco E, Liguori A, Petti F, *et al.* (2008) Traditional acupuncture in migraine: A controlled, randomized study. *Headache* **48(3):** 398–407.

A31 杨雄庆. (2013) 针刺对偏头痛的临床疗效观察. 浙江中医药大学学报 **37(5):** 617–619.

A32 张丽文. (2016) 少阳经穴为主针刺治疗偏头痛 52 例的临床效果. 临床医学研究与实践 **1(9):** 59, 70.

A33 章海凤, 常小荣, 刘密, 刘未艾. (2013) 针刺少阳经特定穴对偏头痛患者近期 VAS 评分头痛强度及 MSQ 评分的临床观察. 时珍国医国药 **24(7):** 1663–1665.

(Continued)

(*Continued*)

A34 赵宗仙. (2014) 龙虎交战镇痛针法治疗偏头痛临床观察. 中国中医药信息杂志 **21(7):** 109–110.

A35 郑光宪. (2015) 针灸联合氟哌噻吨美利曲辛片治疗偏头痛的临床效果观察. 中国当代医药 **22(17):** 149–151.

A36 Linde K, Streng A, Jürgens S, *et al.* (2005) Acupuncture for patients with migraine: A randomized controlled trial. *JAMA* **293(17):** 2118–2125.

A37 Zhao L, Chen J, Li Y, *et al.* (2017) The long-term effect of acupuncture for migraine prophylaxis: A randomized clinical trial. *JAMA Intern Med* **177(4):** 508–515.

A38 Wallasch TM, Weinschuetz T, Mueller B, Kropp P. (2012) Cerebrovascular response in migraineurs during prophylactic treatment with acupuncture: A randomized controlled trial. *J Altern Complement Med* **18(8):** 777–783.

A39 Wang LP, Zhang XZ, Guo J, *et al.* (2011) Efficacy of acupuncture for migraine prophylaxis: A single-blinded, double-dummy, randomized controlled trial. *Pain* **152(8):** 1864–1871.

A40 Wang Y, Xue CC, Helme R, *et al.* (2015) Acupuncture for frequent migraine: A randomized, patient/assessor blinded, controlled trial with one-year follow-up. *Evid Based Complement Alternat Med* **2015:** 920353.

A41 邓竹青. (2012) 针刺少阳经特定穴对偏头痛急性发作期的临床评价研究 (Thesis). 成都中医药大学.

A42 张慧, 胡幼平, 吴佳, 郑晖. (2015) 电针少阳经穴对急性偏头痛即时镇痛作用时效规律研究. 中国针灸 **35(2):** 127–131.

A43 邓启龙. (2012) 头穴透刺治疗偏头痛急性发作疗效观察. 中国中医急症 **21(12):** 2005–2006.

A44 蒋蕾. (2010) 电针太阳穴治疗偏头痛 (肝阳上亢证) 的即时镇痛效应研究 (Thesis). 泸州医学院.

A45 李桂敏, 严伟, 殷建权. (2010) 针刺治疗偏头痛急性发作疗效观察. 上海针灸杂志 **29(07):** 439–441.

A46 任亚东. (2012) 四关穴配曲鬓透率 7 谷治疗 56 例偏头痛即时疗效观察. 四川中医 **30(06):** 113–115.

A47 王赟芝. (2015) 针刺治疗偏头痛缓解后再发疗效观察. 上海针灸杂志 **34(7):** 618–619.

A48 闫国平, 王小霞, 徐晴, 曲国良. (2016) 穴位热痛刺激治疗无先兆偏头痛患者的即时镇痛疗效观察. 中华物理医学与康复杂志 **38(10):** 760–763.

A49 张小泉. (2009) 透刺少阳经头部腧穴治疗偏头痛疗效观察 (Thesis). 广州中医药大学.

A50 Li Y, Liang F, Yang X, *et al.* (2009) Acupuncture for treating acute attacks of migraine: A randomized controlled trial. *Headache* **49(6):** 805–816.

8

Clinical Evidence for Chinese Medicine Combination Therapies

OVERVIEW

Clinical practice of Chinese medicine often sees several therapy types used in combination, such as Chinese herbal medicine plus acupuncture. This chapter presents the evidence of using multiple Chinese medicine therapies to manage migraine. Six randomised controlled trials and two non-randomised controlled trials are included in the evaluation.

Introduction

The practice of using two or more Chinese medicine (CM) interventions such as acupuncture and Chinese herbal medicine (CHM) together is common in clinical management of chronic diseases. In this chapter, randomised controlled trials (RCTs) and non-randomised controlled trials (CCTs) of CM combination therapies were identified and evaluated. There were no non-controlled studies meeting our selection criteria. Previous systematic reviews of CM combination therapies for migraine were not located.

Identification of Clinical Studies

Search of nine English- and Chinese-language databases identified 15,442 citations, of which 449 required full-text retrieval to determine eligibility for inclusion (Fig. 8.1). After assessment against

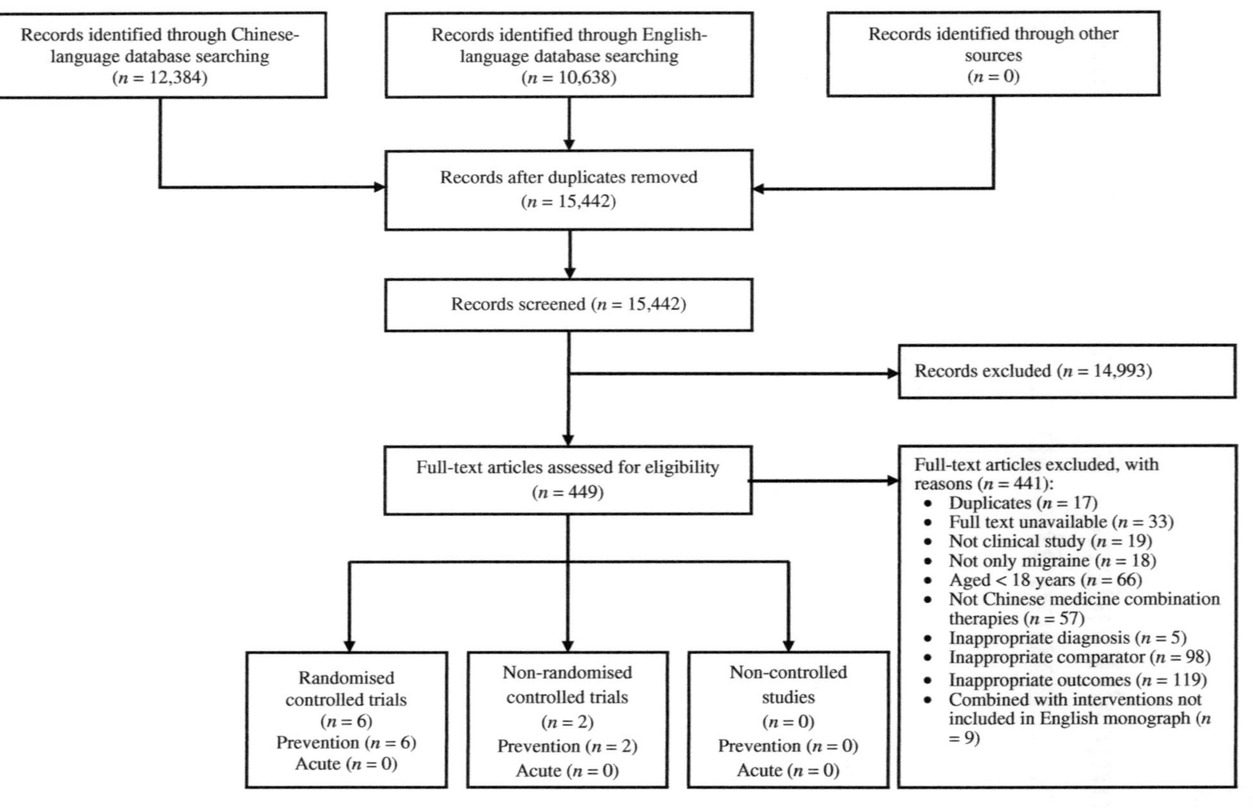

Fig. 8.1. Flowchart of study selection process: Chinese medicine combination therapies

rigorous inclusion criteria, six RCTs (C1–C6) and two CCTs (C7, C8) were included in our evaluation (Fig. 8.1).

In addition, there were three RCTs that applied a combination of CM therapies which are not commonly practised outside China; they are not discussed in this chapter.

The included studies evaluated CM combination therapies as the preventive treatment for migraine. All these studies were conducted in hospitals in China, with 621 participants included in the RCTs and 136 participants involved in the CCTs. More females were included in these studies (female versus male: 454 versus 303, respectively) and the average age of participants was 37.36 years. The duration of migraine was 9.7 years in average. All these studies conducted treatment for four weeks or one month; none of them had a follow-up phase. Chinese medicine syndrome differentiation was not used in these studies.

Therapies used in these studies were CHM, acupuncture, cupping therapy and *tuina* 推拿 therapy. Studies were grouped in four categories; the most common one is CHM plus acupuncture which was tested in five RCTs. See Table 8.1 for a summary.

The most commonly used therapy was acupuncture, which was evaluated by seven studies (C1 to C7); followed by CHM being applied in five studies (C1–C5).

Among all studies, the names of points used for acupuncture or acupressure were provided by six studies. Of the CHM therapies, formula names and herb ingredients were provided by four studies. It is worth pointing out that, although two formulas were named similarly, the actual ingredients of these two formulas are different: *Ju*

Table 8.1. Summary of Interventions in Chinese Medicine Combination Therapies Studies

Combination Therapies	No. of Studies	Included Studies
CHM + acupuncture	5	C1–C5
Acupuncture + mobile cupping	1	C6
Acupuncture + *tuina* 推拿 therapy	1	C7
Acupressure + *tuina* 推拿 therapy	1	C8

Table 8.2. Frequently Reported Herbs in Chinese Medicine Combination Therapies Clinical Studies

Most Common Herbs	Scientific Name	Frequency of Use
Xi xin 细辛	1. *Asarum heterotropoides* Fr. Schmidt var. *mandshuricum* (Maxim) Kitag. 2. *Asarum sieboldii* Miq. var. *seoulense* Nakai 3. *Asarum sieboldii* Miq.	3
Jiang can 僵蚕	1. *Bombyx mori* L. 2. *Beauveria bassiana* (Bals.)	2
Chuan xiong 川芎	*Ligusticum chuangxiong* Hort.	2
Gan cao 甘草	*Glycyrrhiza uralensis* Fisch./ *Glycyrrhiza inflata* Bat./*Glycyrrhiza glabra* L.	2
Bai zhi 白芷	*Angelica dahurica* (Fisch. ex Hoffm.) Benth. et Hook. f.	2

The use of some herbs may be restricted in some countries. Readers are advised to comply with relevant regulations.

Table 8.3. Frequently Used Points/Treatment Approaches in Chinese Medicine Combination Therapies Clinical Studies

Most Common Points	Frequency of Use
GB8 *Shuaigu* 率谷	5
LR3 *Taichong* 太冲	4
EX-HN5 *Taiyang* 太阳	4
GB20 *Fengchi* 风池	4
LI4 *Hegu* 合谷	2
ST8 *Touwei* 头维	2

hua cha tiao san 菊花茶调散 (C3) and *Chuan xiong cha tiao san* 川芎茶调散 (C5).

A total of 22 herbs were used in these formulas. Only five herbs have been used by multiple studies (see Table 8.2). In terms of acupuncture points, 23 points were reported, being used to prevent migraine, with six points being used by multiple studies (see Table 8.3).

Table 8.4.   Risk of Bias Assessment of Randomised Controlled Trials

Risk of Bias Domain	Low Risk *n* (%)	Unclear Risk *n* (%)	High Risk *n* (%)
Sequence generation	1(16.7)	5(83.3)	0(0)
Allocation concealment	0(0)	6(100)	0(0)
Blinding of participants	0(0)	0(0)	6(100)
Blinding of personnel	0(0)	0(0)	6(100)
Blinding of outcome assessor	0(0)	0(0)	6(100)
Incomplete outcome assessment	6(100)	0(0)	0(0)
Selective reporting	0(0)	6(100)	0(0)

Risk of Bias

All included studies were described as RCTs ($n = 6$); only one of them stated an appropriate method for randomisation sequence generation and therefore was assessed as 'low' risk of bias for this domain; the remaining studies were 'unclear' risk due to lack of information. For allocation concealment, all six studies were 'unclear' risk due to lack of information. Blinding of participants, personnel and outcome measures was judged as 'high' risk of bias in all studies because they were all designed to compare different treatments without any effort of blinding. Incomplete outcome data was assessed as 'low' risk of bias for all studies since there were no drop-outs nor missing data. All six studies were 'unclear' risk for selective reporting as protocols could not be identified for the studies. Overall the methodological quality was 'low', so results should be interpreted with caution. See Table 8.4 for a summary.

Chinese Herbal Medicine plus Acupuncture for Migraine Prevention

Randomised Controlled Trials of Chinese Herbal Medicine plus Acupuncture

Five RCTs (C1–C5) evaluated the combination of oral CHM and acupuncture to prevent migraine using pharmacotherapy (flunarizine) as the comparator. Treatment duration was for four weeks or

Table 8.5. Meta-analyses Results: Chinese Herbal Medicine plus Acupuncture versus Flunarizine

Outcome Measure	No. of Studies	No. of Participants	Effect Size (MD [95% CI], I^2)	Included Studies
Migraine frequency, end of treatment	3	299	−3.27 [−7.03, 0.49], 97%	C2, C4, C5
Migraine duration, end of treatment	2	187	−2.04 [−2.54, −1.54]*, 26%	C2, C4
Pain VAS, end of treatment	3	364	−2.20 [−2.47, −1.92]*, 90%	C1, C3, C5

*Statistically significant.

Abbreviations: CI, confidence interval; MD, mean difference; VAS, visual analogue scale.

one month. Among these, CHM formula names were provided by four RCTs: *Shao yao gan cao tang* 芍药甘草汤 (C1), *Ju hua cha tiao san* 菊花茶调散 (C3), *Tong qiao huo xue tang* 通窍活血汤 (C4) and *Chuan xiong cha tiao san* 川芎茶调散 (C5). Acupuncture was administered once a day.

Three studies (C2, C4, C5) reported migraine frequency at the end-of-treatment phase, comparing the combination of oral CHM and acupuncture to flunarizine. Meta-analysis showed there were no significant difference between CM combination therapies and flunarizine (Table 8.5).

Two studies (C2, C4) reported data of migraine duration at the end-of-treatment phase. Meta-analysis showed that the CM combination therapies had significant effects in terms of reducing the monthly migraine duration compared to pharmacotherapy (Table 8.5). In addition, three studies (C1, C3, C5) reported data on pain visual analogue scales (VAS) at the end-of-treatment phase. It was shown by meta-analysis that the CM combination therapies was more effective than flunarizine for pain relief (Table 8.5).

Acupuncture plus Mobile Cupping for Migraine Prevention

One RCT (C6) assessed the treatment of acupuncture in combination with mobile cupping. A total of 70 participants were included in this study. Acupuncture was administered once a day on points including TE23 *Sizhukong* 丝竹空, GB8 *Shuaigu* 率谷, TE5 *Waiguan* 外关 and GB41 *Zulinqi* 足临泣. Mobile cupping on the shoulder and neck region was applied once a week.

Results of this study showed that after applying the combination of acupuncture and mobile cupping for one month, the CM combination therapy was more effective than flunarizine for the outcomes of pain VAS and two domains of Migraine-specific Quality-of-life Questionnaire (MSQ). These results were not confirmed by meta-analysis.

Acupuncture plus *Tuina* 推拿 Therapy

One retrospective trial (C7) compared the combination of acupuncture and *tuina* 推拿 therapy to flunarizine; 96 participants were included in this study. The treatment duration was four weeks. Acupuncture therapy was applied once a day on both local and distal points. The distal points were selected based on CM syndrome differentiation. Chinese medicine *tuina* 推拿 therapy was applied once a day on local acupuncture points. Data showed that, after one month's treatment, the combination of acupuncture and *tuina* 推拿 therapy was more effective for migraine frequency and duration. These results were not confirmed by meta-analysis.

Acupressure plus *Tuina* 推拿 Therapy

One non-randomised controlled trial (C8) compared the combination of acupressure, head *tuina* 推拿 therapy and flunarizine to flunarizine alone; 40 participants were included in this study. The treatment duration was one month. Acupressure was applied twice a week on the points EX-HN5 *Taiyang* 太阳, TE20 *Jiaosun* 角孙, ST8 *Touwei* 头维, GB7 *Qubin* 曲鬓, GB8 *Shuaigu* 率谷 and GB20 *Fengchi* 风池. Head *tuina* 推拿 therapy was also applied two times a day with a simple method: using a comb to massage the scalp along meridians until a feeling of warmth occurs. The results of this study showed that CM combination therapies had a significant add-on effect for pain relief. These results were not confirmed by meta-analysis.

Safety of Chinese Medicine Combination Therapies

Studies did not provide information of adverse events.

Evidence for Chinese Medicine Combination Therapies Commonly Used in Clinical Practice

Our search found there are a limited number of RCTs which have evaluated the combinations of different CM therapies including oral CHM, acupuncture, acupressure, cupping and *tuina* 推拿 therapy for migraine prevention. Except for cupping, all these therapies were recommended by clinical guidelines or textbooks individually (see Chapter 2 for a summary). Meta-analysis results showed that the combination of oral CHM and acupuncture was more effective than flunarizine for migraine prevention, in terms of reducing the duration and pain of migraine attacks. There is no clinical evidence of CM combination therapies for the management of acute migraine.

In combination with other CM therapies, modified versions of *Cha tiao san* 茶调散 formula have been used in multiple studies. Traditionally, *Cha tiao san* 茶调散 has been suggested to treat headache, so it is not surprising that migraine can also be treated by this formula. However, other oral CHM formulas recommended in Chapter 2 were not evaluated by the studies of CM combination therapies.

Acupuncture, acupressure and *tuina* 推拿 therapy were also recommended in Chapter 2 as migraine prevention treatments. Cupping was not a method being recommended by contemporary literature. Although our evaluation identified one RCT of acupuncture in combination with mobile cupping, the effects could not be confirmed due to the limited number of studies.

When applying acupuncture or *tuina* 推拿 therapy, the points of *Shao yang* 少阳 meridians were commonly used. This approach is the same as what was recommended (see Chapter 2) and what has been used in other clinical trials (see Chapter 7).

Summary of Chinese Medicine Combination Therapies Clinical Evidence

This chapter evaluated the combination of two or more CM therapies used as migraine management. All included studies evaluated CHM therapies for migraine prevention, with a treatment duration of one month. Among all included studies, CHM plus acupuncture was the most commonly used combination and acupuncture was the most common therapy being used by all studies.

Among the studies that investigated the combination of CHM and other therapies, only one named oral CHM formula (*Cha tiao san* 茶调散) was identified. Mobile cupping, acupressure and *tuina* 推拿 therapy were also used but with very low numbers. Acupuncture points of *Shao yang* 少阳 meridians were commonly used by these therapies.

Meta-analyses were only applicable for the combination of oral CHM and acupuncture, showing that the CM combination therapy was more effective than flunarizine for migraine duration and pain VAS. Safety information for CM combination therapies is lacking.

References to Included Studies

C1　李存新, 李霞. (2016) 针刺联合芍药甘草汤治疗偏头痛的临床疗效研究. 实用心脑肺血管病杂志 **24(04):** 155–157.

C2　庞明. (2014) 针药并用治疗偏头痛的临床疗效观察. 内蒙古中医药 **33(19):** 51–52.

C3　孙超群. (2015) 菊花茶调散联合针刺治疗偏头痛 90 例临床观察. 河北中医 **37(11):** 1670–1671.

C4　王云松. (2012) 针药结合从络病论治偏头痛 45 例临床观察. 新中医 **44(5):** 97–98.

C5　徐忠, 杨燊. (2013) 川芎茶调散结合针灸治疗偏头痛的疗效观察. 中国民族民间医药杂志 **22(9):** 77–78.

C6　何谊. (2016) 针刺少阳经穴结合颈肩部走罐治疗偏头痛疗效观察. 针灸临床杂志 **32(11):** 33–35.

C7　但洪映. (2016) 盐酸氟桂利嗪胶囊结合中医针灸推拿治疗偏头痛的疗效分析. 系统医学 **1(08):** 19–21, 27.

C8　刘斯雅, 王燕红. (2016) 用穴位按摩联合梳头疗法对偏头痛患者进行治疗的效果分析. 当代医药论丛 **14(8):** 20–21.

9

Summary of Evidence

OVERVIEW

Chinese medicine therapies have been used to treat migraine-like conditions throughout history. In the recent decades, a significant number of clinical studies have been conducted to evaluate Chinese medicine therapies. Findings from clinical evidence revealed promising benefits of oral Chinese herbal medicine and acupuncture therapies. This chapter provides a 'whole-evidence' analysis in investigating Chinese medicine for the management of migraine. The limitations of the available evidence are discussed and future directions are identified for further clinical and experimental research.

Introduction

Migraine is the most common severe form of primary headache with a global prevalence of around one in seven people.[1] It often occurs over many years or over an individual's whole lifetime.[2] Migraine has been ranked as the seventh most common cause of disability worldwide, rising to the third most common cause in those under 50.[3]

It is estimated that, in 2016, migraine affected 1.04 billion individuals and caused 45.1 million years lived with disability (YLDs) globally.[4] In addition, migraine is more prevalent in females; this is considered to be due to the changes in hormone levels during the menstrual cycle.

The two major subtypes of migraine are (1) Migraine with aura; and (2) migraine without aura. Based on the frequency and duration of headaches, migraine can be classified as episodic migraine and chronic migraine. This book focuses on the management of episodic migraine (with aura or without aura), including treatment for acute migraine attacks and prevention treatment.

There is broad variability in the clinical presentation of migraine. Headache attacks vary in intensity of pain and in patterns of associated symptoms. Photophobia, phonophobia, nausea, vomiting, osmophobia and movement sensitivity occur in various combinations. Auras, characterised by visual symptoms (spots of light, zigzag lines or greying out of vision), sensory symptoms (tingling and numbness) or language disturbances occur in 20–30% of people with migraine.[2] Migraine can also present with other types of neurological symptoms; dizziness or vertigo is fairly common in migraine attacks.

Migraine attacks can be triggered by various factors, including dietary factors, menstrual changes, weather, sensory stimuli and stress. However, to some extent, it is challenging to distinguish between migraine triggers and premonitory symptoms which occur two to 48 hours prior to migraine.

The conventional management of migraine consists of two major aspects: prevention of migraine attacks and aborting the acute migraine attacks. In addition to pharmacologic treatments recommended by clinical guidelines and changing lifestyle to avoid triggers, some medical devices and complementary therapies can also be considered.

Chinese medicine (CM) therapies play an important role in the management of migraine, either to assist conventional therapies or to be used alone. In order to provide a 'whole-evidence' evaluation, in this book we analysed the evidence of CM therapies from all types of literature for migraine treatments.

A review of clinical guidelines and textbooks identified a range of CM treatments that have been recommended or suggested for migraine including Chinese herbal medicine (CHM), acupuncture-related therapies and *tuina* 推拿 therapy (Chapter 2).

The disease name 'migraine' in Chinese language is *pian tou tong* 偏头痛, which refers to headaches that occur on one side of the head, describing the main feature of this condition. Considering it is not necessary that migraine headaches only occur on one side of the head, we identified migraine-like conditions from all descriptions of headache recorded in classical literature (Chapter 3). Numerous clinical trials of CM therapies for the treatment of migraine have been conducted in China. Some of these studies have shown promising results. Using a systematic review approach, clinical evidence was found to support the use of oral CHM (Chapter 5) and acupuncture therapy (Chapter 7), and some combination of multiple CM therapies (Chapter 8). The herbs that were used most frequently in the randomised controlled trials (RCTs) have shown actions in experimental studies which shed light on their probable mechanisms of action (Chapter 6).

It should be pointed out that the current clinical management of episodic migraine consists of prevention treatment and treatment for acute migraine attacks, but the treatments recorded in classical literature appeared to relate to managing acute headaches. This could be explained as the preventive effects of CM therapies were not systematically documented in history.

Chinese Medicine Syndrome Differentiation

In the present clinical guidelines or textbooks (see Chapter 2), the CM syndromes for migraine are mainly Liver *yang* uprising 肝阳上亢, phlegm stagnation in the orifices 痰浊蒙窍, Blood stasis in orifices 瘀血阻窍, *qi* and Blood deficiency 气血亏虚, Liver and Kidney *yin* deficiency 肝肾阴虚 and cold stagnated in the Liver meridian 寒凝肝脉.

Classical literature citations included in our evaluation indicated that, in history, migraine was believed to be caused by a combination of external pathogens (wind, cold, fire and heat) and internal pathogens (phlegm and *qi*). The meridian-determined pain location identification also plays an important role in migraine's syndrome differentiation (see Chapter 3).

Syndrome differentiation was reported by approximately half of the clinical studies included in our evaluation (see Chapter 5), with the most commonly seen syndrome being Blood stasis 瘀血阻滞 and Liver *yang* uprising 肝阳上亢. Other syndromes mentioned by the included studies were Liver wind 肝风, Blood deficiency 血虚, *qi* deficiency 气虚 and cold stagnation 寒凝.

Comparing the main syndromes introduced in Chapters 2, 3 and 5, it could be seen that the most commonly recorded aetiology for migraine in CM literature has evolved from external pathogens to internal factors. External pathogens (wind, cold, fire and heat) were recorded in classical literature as the causality of migraine-like condition, while the CM syndromes introduced by contemporary literature and evaluated in modern clinical research were mainly about internal pathogens including Blood stasis and Liver *yang* uprising. It should be noted that the meridian-determined pain location identification also plays an important role in migraine's syndrome differentiation. This approach has been consistently recorded in classical literature and modern literature. In current clinical practice, CHM treatments usually work on resolving the pathogenesis based on syndrome differentiation, with the assistance of some herbs leading the therapeutic effects to certain meridians. On the other hand, acupuncture-related therapies may be more targeting particular symptoms in combination with treatment based on meridian-determined syndrome differentiation.

However, although some clinical studies have used syndrome differentiation for treatment selection (especially if multiple formulas were used in the study), results are usually reported in aggregate and not by syndrome type. Hence it was not possible to conduct sub-group analyses based on syndrome type to establish efficacy of treatments according to specific syndromes.

Chinese Herbal Medicine

This section summarises the evidence from Chapters 2, 3, 5 and 8.

Chinese herbal medicine therapies have been suggested by all forms of clinical evidence in the treatment of migraine. Oral CHM has been recommended as the main body of CM therapy by contemporary textbooks and guidelines and also evaluated in clinical studies. Oral CHM has also been recorded in classical literature as the treatment for clinical conditions presenting symptoms likely to be migraine. Topically used CHM has been recommended by clinical guidelines in the forms of sniffing, external application, fumigation and steaming therapy. Chinese herbal medicine sniffing and external application methods were also found in classical literature as the treatment for migraine-like condition; however, there is no clinical research assessing the effects of topically used CHM according to our systematic evaluation.

Since historically migraine's aetiology in CM theory has evolved from external pathogens to internal factors, the treatment principles of CM concepts were also developed from addressing external factors to resolving the internal aetiology. Consequently, the CHM formulas and frequently used herbs recorded in classical literature are not consistent with those used in current clinical practice. For example, the CHM formula *Qing kong gao* 清空膏 is the most frequent oral formula found in classical literature, with clearing wind heat being the key treatment principle. However, this formula is not commonly used for migraine in current clinical practice.

Oral Chinese Herbal Medicine

The analysis of treatment effects showed promising clinical evidence with oral CHM formulas and products, especially for preventing episodic migraine attacks. The evaluation of modern literature evidence showed that, when oral CHM was used as prevention treatment, it was more effective than pharmacotherapy in terms of reducing the frequency of migraine, migraine days, pain of migraine and acute medication usage. On the other hand, when oral CHM was used in addition to pharmacotherapy, it increased the treatment effects of reducing the frequency of migraine, migraine days and pain of migraine. In particular, meta-analysis results support the use of the following oral CHM formulas: *Zheng tian wan* or *Zheng tian jiao nang* 正天丸 (正天胶囊), *Yang xue qing nao ke li* 养血清脑颗粒, *Chuan xiong cha tiao san* 川芎茶调散 and *Jia wei san pian tang* 加味散偏汤.

There were only two RCTs evaluating oral CHM as abortive treatment for acute migraine attacks, without meta-analysis results to confirm the treatment effects. For migraine prevention, in order to provide evidence regarding possibly effective herbs used in clinical practice, the most frequent herbs used in studies from favourable meta-analyses were calculated. Studies were pooled according to four main outcome measures regardless of their comparator: (1) monthly migraine frequency, duration and migraine days, all these being calculated on a monthly base; (2) responder rate; (3) migraine pain visual analogue scale (VAS) or numeric rating scale (NRS); and (4) acute medication usage (see Table 5.9). The most frequently used herbs for each outcome measure are similar. It was found that two herbs, *chuan xiong* 川芎 and *bai zhi* 白芷, were repeatedly shown in all four outcome domains, followed by *dang gui* 当归, *bai shao* 白芍, *xi xin* 细辛, *gan cao* 甘草 and *gou teng* 钩藤 which have been shown in three outcome domains.

The herbs that were frequently used as oral CHM treatments for migraine-like conditions in classical literature are listed in Table 3.12. Among these herbs, nine herbs (*gan cao* 甘草, *chuan xiong* 川芎, *fang feng* 防风, *qiang huo* 羌活, *chai hu* 柴胡, *tian ma* 天麻, *bai zhi* 白芷, *xi xin* 细辛 and *quan xie* 全蝎) were also shown in the list of 'frequently reported orally used herbs in meta-analyses showing favourable effect for migraine' (Table 5.9). However, more than half of these most frequently used herbs were not shown in the list of 'meta-analyses showing favourable effect for migraine', which indicates that there is diversity between what has been recorded in classical literature and those proven effective by clinical research.

Clinical studies have reported the safety of oral CHM, with mild gastrointestinal adverse events being associated with CHM. All these adverse events ceased by adjusting the time and dosage of medicine and no additional medical attention was required.

However, certain heterogeneity in meta-analyses indicates that there was considerable variability in each result. At least part of this variability was due to the use of different CHMs, but it was not possible for us to determine which CHM produced the greatest effects since most studies tested different formulas even though many were based on similar ingredients. Other factors influencing the interpretation of the results of the clinical studies were the relatively poor reporting of trial design and methods and the lack of blinding in most studies. These aspects reduced confidence in the accuracy of the reported results and influenced the downgrading of the quality of the evidence in the Grading of Recommendations Assessment, Development and Evaluation (GRADE) assessments.

Chinese Herbal Medicine Formulas in Key Clinical Guidelines and Textbooks, Classical Literature and Clinical Studies

Table 9.1 summarises the oral CHM formulas described in clinical guidelines and textbooks (Chapter 2), classical literature (Chapter 3) and clinical studies (Chapter 5). Assessment was based on formula name. It is likely that formulas with the same, or similar, herb ingredients but with different formula names were also included in classical literature and clinical research. As assessment of similarity of formulas is complex and was not undertaken, the actual number for each listed formula may be higher than reported below.

Based on our analysis, the formulas recorded in classical literature are not completely consistent with those being commonly used in current clinical practice. None of the CHM formulas were seen in all forms of literature (classical literature, contemporary textbooks/clinical guidelines and clinical research).

Wu zhu yu tang 吴茱萸汤 is the only oral CHM formula that was identified from classical literature and also recommended by current clinical guidelines/textbooks. *Cha tiao san* 茶调散, *Chuan xiong cha tiao san* 川芎茶调散 and *Ju hua cha tiao san* 菊花茶调散 share similar names and ingredients. They were developed in the long history of CHM clinical practice based on similar treatment principles. Among these three formulas, *Cha tiao san* 茶调散 and *Chuan xiong cha tiao san* 川芎茶调散 have certain evidence from classical literature, while *Ju hua cha tiao san* 菊花茶调散 is evidenced in modern clinical research. *Zheng tian wan* 正天丸 and *Yang xue qing nao ke li* 养血清脑颗粒 are two CHM products recommended by current clinical guidelines/textbooks, as well as evaluated by clinical research. Among these formulas, only *Yang xue qing nao ke li* 养血清脑颗粒 has been evaluated as a treatment for acute migraine management by one RCT (see Table 9.1).

Table 9.1. Summary of Oral Chinese Herbal Medicine Formulas

Formula Name	Evidence in Clinical Guidelines and Textbooks (Chapter 2)	Evidence in Classical Literature (No. of Citations)	Included in Clinical Studies (No. of Studies) (Chapter 5)			Included in Combination Therapies (No. of Studies) (Chapter 8)
			RCTs	CCTs	Non-controlled Studies	
Tian ma gou teng yin 天麻钩藤饮	Yes	0	0	0	0	0
Ban xia bai zhu tian ma tang 半夏白术天麻汤	Yes	0	0	0	0	0
Tong qiao huo xue tang 通窍活血汤	Yes	0	0	0	0	1
Ba zhen tang 八珍汤	Yes	0	0	0	0	0
Qi ju di huang wan 杞菊地黄丸	Yes	0	0	0	0	0
Wu zhu yu tang 吴茱萸汤	Yes	10	0	0	0	0
Tong tian oral solution 通天口服液	Yes	0	0	0	0	0
Quan tian ma capsule 全天麻胶囊	Yes	0	0	0	0	0
Zheng tian wan 正天丸	Yes	0	5	1	0	0

Fu fang yang jiao pian 复方羊角片 or *Fu fang yang jiao ke li* 复方羊角颗粒	Yes	0	0	0	0	0
Xue fu zhu yu oral solution 血府逐瘀口服液	Yes	0	0	0	0	0
Yang xue qing nao ke li 养血清脑颗粒	Yes	0	5	0	1	0
Tian ma tou tong tablet 天麻头痛片	Yes	0	0	0	0	0
Qing kong gao 清空膏	No	17	0	0	0	0
Zhui feng san 追风散	No	7	0	0	0	0
Ru xiang zhan luo san 乳香盏落散	No	6	0	0	0	0
Ru sheng bing zi 如圣饼子	No	6	0	0	0	0
Ren shen ban xia wan 人参半夏丸	No	5	0	0	0	0
Xiong xin tang 芎辛汤	No	4	0	0	0	0
Da fu wan 大附丸	No	2	0	0	0	0

(*Continued*)

Table 9.1. (*Continued*)

Formula Name	Evidence in Clinical Guidelines and Textbooks (Chapter 2)	Evidence in Classical Literature (No. of Citations)	Included in Clinical Studies (No. of Studies) (Chapter 5)			Included in Combination Therapies (No. of Studies) (Chapter 8)
			RCTs	CCTs	Non-controlled Studies	
Tai yi zi jin dan 太乙紫金丹	No	2	0	0	0	0
Bi sheng san 必胜散	No	2	0	0	0	0
Shi gao wan 石膏丸	No	2	0	0	0	0
Kong qing gao 空青膏	No	2	0	0	0	0
Cha tiao san 茶调散	No	2	0	0	0	0
Huang niu nao sui jiu 黄牛脑髓酒	No	2	0	0	0	0
Chuan xiong cha tiao san 川芎茶调散	No	0	3	0	0	1
Ju hua cha tiao san 菊花茶调散						
Tou ding san 透顶散	No	11	0	0	0	0
Tong ding san 通顶散	No	3	0	0	0	0
Long xiang san 龙香散	No	3	0	0	0	0
San pian tang 散偏汤	No	0	2	0	0	0
Chai shao zhi tong fang 柴芍止痛方	No	0	2	0	0	0

Abbreviations: CCTs, controlled clinical trials; RCTs, randomised controlled trials.

Except for these four CHM formulas, there are many CHM formulas only shown in one type of evidence (classical literature, contemporary literature or modern clinical research literature) (see Table 9.1). A few factors may have contributed to such inconsistency; they are: (1) The historical development of migraine's aetiology in the concept of CM leads to the change of treatment principles and formulas; (2) During the evolvement of CM theory and formulas over two thousand years, some of the CHM formulas used in current clinical practice are modified versions of certain formulas but named differently.

It should be pointed out that although the oral CHM formula *Chuan xiong cha tiao san* 川芎茶调散 is often used in clinical practice to treat headaches, and multiple clinical studies included in this research evaluated the effects of this formula, it is neither shown in the 'most likely' migraine citations of classical literature, nor recommended by current clinical guidelines as migraine treatment.

Topical Chinese Herbal Medicine

Topically used CHM therapies were recommended by clinical guidelines in the forms of sniffing, external application, fumigation and steaming therapy (see Chapter 2 for details). Most of the topical CHM therapies used unnamed CHM formulas. Our evaluation of classical literature identified three CHM formulas used as topical CHM therapy; they were: *Tou ding san* 透顶散, *Tong ding san* 通顶散 and *Long xiang san* 龙香散 (Table 3.11). These formulas were recorded being used as sniffing or external application. However, there is no clinical study included in our evaluation of the modern literature and therefore the effects of topical CHM for migraine cannot be confirmed. See Table 9.2 for a summary.

Acupuncture-related and Other Chinese Medicine Therapies

This section summarises the evidence from Chapters 2, 3, 7 and 8.

Acupuncture therapies have a long history of use for the clinical management of symptoms likely to be migraine. According to our evaluation, acupuncture treatment (referring to the traditional style of

Table 9.2. Summary of Topical Chinese Herbal Medicine Formulas

Formula Name	Evidence in Clinical Guidelines and Textbooks (Chapter 2)	Evidence in Classical Literature (No. of Citations)	Included in Clinical Studies (No. of Studies) (Chapter 5)			Included in Combination Therapies (No. of Studies) (Chapter 8)
			RCTs	CCTs	Non-controlled Studies	
Chu bi san 搐鼻散	Yes	0	0	0	0	0
CHM external application: *Di long* 地龙, *quan xie* 全蝎, *lu lu tong* 路路通, *sheng nan xing* 生南星, *sheng ban xia* 生半夏, *bai fu zi* 白附子 and *xi xin* 细辛	Yes	0	0	0	0	0
CHM fumigation and steaming therapy: *Xi xin* 细辛, *shi chang pu* 石菖蒲, *qiang huo* 羌活, *zi su* 紫苏, *chuan xiong* 川芎 and *jiang can* 僵蚕	Yes	0	0	0	0	0
Tou ding san 透顶散	No	11	0	0	0	0
Tong ding san 通顶散	No	3	0	0	0	0
Long xiang san 龙香散	No	3	0	0	0	0

Abbreviations: CCTs, controlled clinical trials; CHM, Chinese herbal medicine; RCTs, randomised controlled trials.

body acupuncture) has been recommended by textbooks and clinical guidelines, and recorded as an effective therapy in classical literature, as well as been intensively researched by clinical studies. Acupuncture seems an effective treatment for preventing migraine attacks, as well as managing acute migraine.

Moxibustion has all forms of evidence also; however, with a very small number of clinical studies. Two modern forms of acupuncture developed based on the theory of reflexology (scalp acupuncture and ear acupressure), also have been recommended by contemporary literature and researched by clinical studies. *Tuina* 推拿 therapy is one of the clinical guideline-recommended therapies. However, it is not identified from classical literature, and clinical research on *tuina* 推拿 therapy alone is lacking. See Table 9.3 for a detailed summary of these therapies across different types of literature.

In order to summarise which acupuncture points were used for acupuncture-related treatment, the points that were recommended in Chapter 2 and used in the RCTs in Chapter 7 and Chapter 8 are presented in Table 9.4. The use of these points was cross-referenced to

Table 9.3. Summary of Acupuncture-related and Other Therapies

Therapies	Included in Clinical Guidelines and Textbooks (Chapter 2)	Included in Classical Literature (Chapter 3) (No. of Citations)	Included in Clinical Studies (No. of Studies) (Chapter 7)			Included in Combination Therapies (No. of Studies) (Chapter 8)
			RCTs*	CCTs*	Non-controlled Studies*	
Body acupuncture	Yes	4	47	0	0	8
Scalp acupuncture	Yes	0	3	0	0	0
Moxibustion	Yes	4	1	0	0	0
Ear acupressure	Yes	0	2	0	0	0
Tuina 推拿 therapy	Yes	0	0	0	0	2

*Some studies used more than one intervention e.g. acupuncture plus moxibustion. These are counted separately in this table.

Abbreviations: CCTs, controlled clinical trials; RCTs, randomised controlled trials.

Table 9.4.   Summary of Acupuncture Points

Acupuncture Point	Clinical Guidelines and Textbooks (Chapter 2)	Classical Literature (Chapter 3) (No. of Citations)	Clinical Studies (No. of Studies) (Chapter 7)			Combination Therapies (No. of Studies) (Chapter 8)
			RCTs	CCTs	Non-controlled Studies*	
Acupuncture						
TE23 *Sizhukong* 丝竹空	Yes	0	6	0	0	1
GB8 *Shuaigu* 率谷	Yes	5	27	0	0	5
EX-HN5 *Taiyang* 太阳	Yes	0	20	0	0	4
GB20 *Fengchi* 风池	Yes	2	29	0	0	4
LI4 *Hegu* 合谷	Yes	0	13	0	0	2
LR3 *Taichong* 太冲	Yes	0	13	0	0	4
GB41 *Zulinqi* 足临泣	Yes	0	9	0	0	1
GB34 *Yanglingquan* 阳陵泉	Yes	0	17	0	0	0
TE5 *Waiguan* 外关	Yes	0	19	0	0	1
GB4 *Hanyan* 颔厌	Yes	0	0	0	0	0
GB5 *Xuanlu* 悬颅	Yes	0	0	0	0	0
LU7 *Lieque* 列缺	Yes	0	0	0	0	0
KI3 *Taixi* 太溪	Yes	0	0	0	0	0
LR2 *Xingjian* 行间	Yes	0	0	0	0	0
ST40 *Fenglong* 丰隆	Yes	0	0	0	0	0
PC6 *Neiguan* 内关	Yes	0	0	0	0	0
BL17 *Geshu* 膈俞	Yes	0	0	0	0	0
SP10 *Xuehai* 血海	Yes	0	0	0	0	0
ST36 *Zusanli* 足三里	Yes	0	0	0	0	0
SP6 *Sanyinjiao* 三阴交	Yes	0	0	0	0	0
CV6 *Qihai* 气海	Yes	0	0	0	0	0
BL23 *Shenshu* 肾俞	Yes	0	0	0	0	0
GV26 *Shuigou* 水沟	Yes	0	1	0	0	0
HT7 *Shenmen* 神门	Yes	0	0	0	0	0
GV20 *Baihui* 百会	Yes	0	12	0	0	0
ST8 *Touwei* 头维	Yes	2	7	0	0	0
BL10 *Tianzhu* 天柱	Yes	0	0	0	0	0

Table 9.4.   (*Continued*)

Acupuncture Point	Clinical Guidelines and Textbooks (Chapter 2)	Classical Literature (Chapter 3) (No. of Citations)	Clinical Studies (No. of Studies) (Chapter 7)			Combination Therapies (No. of Studies) (Chapter 8)
			RCTs	CCTs	Non-controlled Studies*	
GB13 *Benshen* 本神	No	2	0	0	0	0
GB40 *Qiuxu* 丘墟	No	0	13	0	0	0
TE20 *Jiaosun* 角孙	No	0	10	0	0	0
Ashi 阿是穴	No	0	6	0	0	0
BL60 *Kunlun* 昆仑	No	0	5	0	0	0
Scalp Acupuncture 头皮针						
GV21 *Qianding* 前顶	Yes	0	0	0	0	0
MS8 顶旁 I 线	Yes	0	0	0	0	0
MS9 顶旁 II 线	Yes	0	0	0	0	0
MS10 颞前线	No	0	2	0	0	0
MS11 颞后线	No	0	2	0	0	0
Ear Acupuncture and Ear Acupressure						
TF4 *Shenmen* 神门	Yes	0	2	0	0	0
AT4 *Subcotex* 皮质下	Yes	0	2	0	0	0
AT3 *Occiput* 枕	Yes	0	2	0	0	0
AT1 *Forehead* 额	Yes	0	2	0	0	0
AH6a *Sympathetic* 交感	No	0	2	0	0	0
Moxibustion						
EX-HN5 *Taiyang* 太阳	Yes	0	1	0	0	0
GB20 *Fengchi* 风池	Yes	0	1	0	0	0
GV20 *Baihui* 百会	Yes	0	0	0	0	0
GB8 *Shuaigu* 率谷	Yes	0	1	0	0	0
GB22 *Xinhui* 囟会	Yes	0	0	0	0	0
EX-HN3 *Yintang* 印堂	Yes	0	1	0	0	0
LR2 *Xingjian* 行间	Yes	0	0	0	0	0
BL10 *Tianzhu* 天柱	Yes	0	0	0	0	0
TE5 *Waiguan* 外关	Yes	0	1	0	0	0

(*Continued*)

Table 9.4.   (*Continued*)

Acupuncture Point	Clinical Guidelines and Textbooks (Chapter 2)	Classical Literature (Chapter 3) (No. of Citations)	Clinical Studies (No. of Studies) (Chapter 7)			Combination Therapies (No. of Studies) (Chapter 8)
			RCTs	CCTs	Non-controlled Studies*	
***Tuina* 推拿 Therapy**						
EX-HN3 *Yintang* 印堂	Yes	0	0	0	0	1
EX-HN5 *Taiyang* 太阳	Yes	0	0	0	0	1
GV20 *Baihui* 百会	Yes	0	0	0	0	1
GB20 *Fengchi* 风池	Yes	0	0	0	0	1
BL1 *Jingming* 睛明	Yes	0	0	0	0	0
ST8 *Touwei* 头维	Yes	0	0	0	0	1
LI4 *Hegu* 合谷	Yes	0	0	0	0	0
LI11 *Quchi* 曲池	Yes	0	0	0	0	0
ST36 *Zusanli* 足三里	Yes	0	0	0	0	0
LR2 *Xingjian* 行间	Yes	0	0	0	0	0

*Some studies used more than one intervention e.g. oral Chinese herbal medicine plus moxibustion. These are counted separately in this table.

Abbreviations: CCTs, controlled clinical trials; RCTs, randomised controlled trials.

other clinical trial types and other chapters. According to this summary, for body acupuncture treatment, there are two points that have evidence from all forms of literature (GB8 *Shuaigu* 率谷 and GB20 *Fengchi* 风池), and another seven points that were recommended by contemporary literature, as well as evaluated by clinical studies (TE23 *Sizhukong* 丝竹空, EX-HN5 *Taiyang* 太阳, LI4 *Hegu* 合谷, LR3 *Taichong* 太冲, GB41 *Zulinqi* 足临泣, GB34 *Yanglingquan* 阳陵泉 and TE5 *Waiguan* 外关). All these points were also shown in the list of 'Frequently Reported Acupuncture Points in Meta-analyses Showing Favourable Effect for Migraine Prevention' (Table 7.9). Five points (GB8 *Shuaigu* 率谷, GB20 *Fengchi* 风池, EX-HN5 *Taiyang* 太阳, GB34 *Yanglingquan* 阳陵泉 and TE5 *Waiguan* 外关) were also shown in the list of 'Frequently Reported Acupuncture Points in Meta-analyses Showing Favourable Effect for Acute Migraine Management' (Table 7.15). This consistency indicates the effectiveness of acupuncture treatment for both migraine prevention and acute management. It should be noted that only four acupuncture points were identified from multiple citations of the classical literature evaluation; these were GB8 *Shuaigu* 率谷 (*n* = 3), ST8 *Touwei* 头维 (*n* = 2), GB13 *Benshen* 本神 (*n* = 2) and GB20 *Fengchi* 风池 (*n* = 2). In fact, we identified classical literature citations which were 'possibly' referring to migraine-like conditions, but there were only ten citations which were included in the 'most likely' migraine pool, due to the lack of detailed descriptions of disease recorded in those acupuncture citations. This is caused by the fact that, in classical literature, the records of acupuncture therapies were usually from the angle of introducing the function of points rather than from the angle of a disease. Furthermore, the clinical evidence of moxibustion, scalp acupuncture, ear acupressure and *tuina* 推拿 therapy are not convincing due to the very small number of studies included in this research.

It is worth noting that the points from the Gallbladder meridian are commonly selected for the management of migraine. This could be explained by two reasons: (1) The location of migraine is usually dominated by the Gallbladder meridian; and (2) The CM syndrome of migraine is related to Liver/Gallbladder abnormalities.

Limitations of the Evidence

Certain limitations should be noted from each of the data sources, in particular the classical literature. Firstly, analyses of the classical literature (Chapter 3) was based on the large sample of CM books included in the *Zhong Hua Yi Dian* 中华医典 version 5. Our assessments indicated that this was the largest available digital resource at the time, but it did not include every CM book published in premodern eras so omissions are inevitable.

Secondly, although there was a large amount of information about treatments for headaches recorded in classical books, the specific condition migraine was not easy to be differentiated from other types of headache. The currently used disease name, *pian tou tong* 偏头痛 (referring to migraine in the Chinese language), means 'headache occurring on one side of the head'. However, it is not necessary that migraine only presents as one-sided headache. Therefore, we could not simply rely on words such as *pian* 偏, *ban* 半, or *ban bian* 半边 to identify migraine-like conditions. The approach we used to identify relevant citations in classical literature was to firstly, include all types of headaches, then select the citations which also described typical migraine symptoms using a scoring method (see Table 3.2). The final pool of 'most likely' migraine citations was limited to those citations with a score greater than three. This approach ensured the accuracy of the citations included in the final pool; however, we could not be certain that all relevant citations were located and included in our analyses since the classical books have not always described detailed symptoms together with the treatments. Thirdly, it is not accurate to assume that the most frequently used herbs represent the most effective treatments because there is no method to evaluate the efficacy. What they represent is a short list of herbs that could be considered for further research.

The clinical trial evidence was based on searches of multiple databases and resulted in thousands of search results. Since there was considerable variation in the conditions under which these trials were conducted, the age and severity of the participants, the frequency and duration of interventions and the procedures used in data collection and analysis, it was not surprising that statistical heterogeneity tended to be 'high' in some meta-analyses, although random effects models were used. The quality of the reporting of the methodological details of trial design and conduct was not adequate in many studies.

For the clinical studies evaluating the effects of CHM, only a small proportion of studies involved placebo CHM and therefore they may achieve blinding of participants; other studies all carried the risk of performance bias due to the lack of blinding. Due to the lack of blinding, the efficacy of the results achieved may not reflect the real therapeutic effects of CM therapies, since there have possibly been non-specific effects caused by adding an additional treatment. For the studies that investigated acupuncture-related therapies, the proportion of studies that applied sham control is higher than that of the CHM studies; however, the sham control methods were designed differently.

Furthermore, for each category of evidence, frequency tables are provided that summarise the most commonly used interventions including the herbal formula names, the herbal ingredients used in the formulas and the acupuncture points used in the clinical studies. Due to the large volume of available data, presentation of the details of every study was not feasible and these tables only include the interventions that were the most frequently used. Also, it should not be assumed that the most frequently used interventions were the most effective ones. The above limitations should be taken in consideration when interpreting the results included in the previous chapters.

Implications for Practice

In the traditional context, CM practice is inherited from the records in previous literature or senior practitioners' clinical experience. To date, the evidence-based practice approach was not adopted for the development of textbooks or clinical practice guidelines in CM. In this research, we evaluated evidence from classical literature and current clinical research and provided information of how and to what extent treatments of migraine were developed. The research provides evidence which supports the recommendation for use of CM therapies and identified the gaps between contemporary literature and current clinical practice, in terms of some treatment methods.

There was vast information of treatments for headaches recorded in classical literature. Migraine is a special type of primary headache with unique symptoms. However, migraine was not clearly defined as a specific disease in the long history of CM. Only less than 200 descriptions were identified as 'most likely' migraine treatments, including oral CHM, topical CHM and acupuncture-related therapies. The CHM formulas used in history were not totally consistent with those being used in current clinical practice, but it is worth noting that topical CHM was recorded in classical literature for the treatment of migraine, which seemed more popular in history than the current CM clinical practice. However, the effects of topical CHM need to be confirmed.

Based on our analyses, the following main findings may be considered to apply in clinical practice:

- The CM syndrome differentiation of migraine is mainly Blood stasis 瘀血阻滞 and Liver *yang* uprising 肝阳上亢;
- Meridian-determined syndrome differentiation based on the location of pain plays an important role, particularly in acupuncture-related therapies;
- Oral CHM seems effective for preventing episodic migraine;
- A group of herbs (oral) were found frequently used in classical literature and may be effective according to our analysis of modern clinical research; they are *gan cao* 甘草, *chuan xiong* 川芎, *fang feng* 防风, *qiang huo* 羌活, *chai hu* 柴胡, *tian ma* 天麻, *bai zhi* 白芷, *xi xin* 细辛 and *quan xie* 全蝎;
- Acupuncture seems effective for both episodic migraine prevention and acute migraine treatment;
- Acupuncture points to consider are GB8 *Shuaigu* 率谷, GB20 *Fengchi* 风池, TE23 *Sizhukong* 丝竹空, EX-HN5 *Taiyang* 太阳, LI4 *Hegu* 合谷, LR3 *Taichong* 太冲, GB41 *Zulinqi* 足临泣, GB34 *Yanglingquan* 阳陵泉 and TE5 *Waiguan* 外关.

It should be pointed out that the use of some herbs may be restricted in some countries, for example, *xi xin* 细辛 can be toxic, and some herbs identified from classical literature (e.g. *she xiang* 麝香) may be restricted under the Convention on International Trade in Endangered Species of Wild Fauna and Flora (CITES); readers are advised to comply with relevant regulations.

Using the GRADE approach to assess the certainty of evidence identified from clinical research, it was found that most of the CHM evidence was assessed as 'low' certainty, while the evidence of acupuncture was assessed with higher certainty ('moderate'). Therefore, the interpretation and application of the evidence should be done with caution.

Implications for Research

Chinese medicine therapies are increasingly evaluated through clinical trials, in line with the development of Western medicine. Our systematic analysis found that the CM management of migraine are consistent and encouraging, but high-quality evidence is lacking. Hence, there is a need for well-designed clinical trials of CM interventions in order to provide reliable assessment of treatment effects. Further high-quality clinical trials are needed which addresses the following aspects: (1) general trial design; (2) intervention and control; (3) outcome measures; and (4) reporting.

General Trial Design

- Randomised controlled trials should be designed with rigorous methodology with particular attention paid to adequate randomisation and allocation concealment;
- Clinical studies should evaluate the treatments for acute migraine and prevention of migraine separately;
- When using a clinical practice guideline-recommended therapy as control, the treatment duration should be designed meeting the standard recommended in guidelines;
- Since CM therapies are commonly administered as add-on therapies to routine care, efforts should be made to ensure blinding of participants and practitioner with the use of placebo or sham control;
- Clinical trial protocols should be registered in the Clinical Trial Registry or be published prior to the conduct of RCTs to increase transparency in reporting.

Intervention and Control

- For CHM, authentication of raw material should be described and for manufactured products, reports should include the quantity of active constituents;
- Syndrome differentiation should be considered in the study design to improve applicability in clinical practice;

- Placebo control for CHM should be applied when testing the add-on effects of integrating CHM with routine care, to rule out the potential bias caused by lack of blinding of participants and personnel;
- Topical CHM and some CM therapies commonly used in clinical practice (e.g. *taichi* 太极) have not been researched well enough; future research may consider evaluating the effectiveness of these therapies;
- Although sham control has been applied in recent acupuncture clinical trials, the sham control methods used in these studies were different. It has been acknowledged that an ideal design of a proper placebo acupuncture to ensure double-blinding is challenging.[5,6] Pragmatic trials designed to evaluate the effectiveness of interventions in real-life routine practice conditions will also provide valuable evidence to prove the effects of acupuncture-related therapies.

Outcome Measures

Most of the included clinical studies were conducted in China and published in the Chinese language. Diversity was found in the outcome measures used in clinical research. Regarding prevention of episodic migraine, the most commonly reported outcome measures were the monthly frequency and duration of migraine and pain severity. Health-related quality of life outcome measures were rarely used by the clinical studies included in our evaluation. Future research should pay more attention to assessing the impact of migraine on patients' quality of life, using widely accepted disease-specific health-related quality of life and disability instruments, such as the Migraine Disability Assessment Test (MIDAS), the Headache Impact Test-6 (HIT-6) and the Migraine-specific Quality-of-Life Questionnaire (MSQ).

In addition, since there is a link between migraine and depression/anxiety and an inseparable relationship between sleep and migraine, future studies may consider including outcome measures to evaluate patients' psychological status and sleep quality.

Reporting

- Research reports should follow the CONSORT statement with reference to the extension for herbal medicine[7] and STRICTA for clinical trials of acupuncture;[8]
- Individual modification to the CHM formula or acupuncture points should be reported with more detail in order to instruct real-life clinical practice;
- Any modification or adjustment to the treatment method recommended by current clinical guidelines and the why and how of it, should be addressed when reporting the results;
- Adverse events information should be reported with more detail, and the causality and their relationship with the CM therapy should be addressed.

Diversity was seen in the range of CM therapies, both within and across forms of evidence, reflecting the nature of CM clinical practice. Future research should focus on the most promising findings identified and investigate the efficacy and safety of those therapies that are feasible to be widely used in clinical practice.

The consistency with which certain herbs were used as ingredients in classical formulas (Chapter 3) and in clinical trials (Chapter 5) was highlighted by the herb frequency analyses in each of these chapters. As Chapter 6 briefly summarised, there have been a number of experimental studies on these frequently used herbs which have demonstrated bioactivities that are relevant to migraine and may, at least, partially explain how the herbal formulas could have acted. Future studies could assess the effects of these herbs and their constituent compounds in various combinations as they are commonly used in the formulas.

References

1. Steiner TJ, Stovner LJ, Birbeck GL. (2013) Migraine: The seventh disabler. *J Headache Pain* **14(1):** 1.
2. Headache Classification Committee of the International Headache Society (IHS). (2018) The International Classification of Headache Disorders, 3rd ed. *Cephalalgia* **38(1):** 1–211.

3. Steiner TJ, Stovner LJ, Vos T. (2016) GBD 2015: Migraine is the third cause of disability in under 50s. *J Headache Pain* **17(1):** 104.

4. Saylor D, Steiner TJ. (2018) The global burden of headache. *Semin Neurol* **38(2):** 182–190.

5. Zhang CS, Tan HY, Zhang GS, *et al.* (2015) Placebo devices as effective control methods in acupuncture clinical trials: A systematic review. *PLoS One* **10(11):** e0140825.

6. Zhang GS, Zhang CS, Tan HY, *et al.* (2018) Systematic review of acupuncture placebo devices with a focus on the credibility of blinding of healthy participants and/or acupuncturists. *Acupunct Med* **36(4):** 204–214.

7. Pandis N, Chung B, Scherer RW, *et al.* (2017) CONSORT 2010 statement: Extension checklist for reporting within person randomised trials. *BMJ* **357:** j2835.

8. MacPherson H, White A, Cummings M, *et al.* (2001) Standards for reporting interventions in controlled trials of acupuncture: The STRICTA recommendations. *Complement Ther Med* **9(4):** 246–249.

Glossary

Glossary of Terms	Abbreviation	Definition	Reference
95% confidence interval	95% CI	A measure of the uncertainty around the main finding of a statistical analysis. Estimates of unknown quantities, such as the odds ratio comparing an experimental intervention with a control, are usually presented as a point estimate and a 95% confidence interval. This means that if a study was repeated in other samples from the same population, 95% of the confidence intervals from those studies would contain the true value of the unknown quantity. Alternatives to 95%, such as 90% and 99% confidence intervals, are sometimes used. Wider intervals indicate lower precision; narrow intervals indicate greater precision.	http://handbook.cochrane.org
Acupuncture	—	The insertion of needles into humans or animals for remedial purposes.	World Health Organisation. (2007) WHO International Standard Terminologies of Traditional Medicine in the Western Pacific Region.
Allied and Complementary Medicine Database	AMED	Alternative medicine bibliographic database.	https://www.ebsco.com/products/research-databases/allied-and-complementary-medicine-database-amed

(Continued)

(*Continued*)

Glossary of Terms	Abbreviation	Definition	Reference
Aura	—	Auras are characterised by visual symptoms (spots of light, zigzag lines or greying out of vision), sensory symptoms (tingling and numbness) or language disturbances, which occur in 20–30% of people with migraine.	Headache Classification Committee of the International Headache Society (IHS). (2013) The International Classification of Headache Disorders, 3rd ed. (beta version). *Cephalalgia* **33(9):** 629–808.
China National Knowledge Infrastructure	CNKI	Chinese language bibliographic database.	www.cnki.net
Chinese Biomedical Literature database	CBM	Chinese language bibliographic database.	https://cbmwww.imicams.ac.cn
Chinese herbal medicine	CHM	—	—
Chinese medicine	CM	—	—
Chongqing VIP Information Company	CQVIP	Chinese-language bibliographic database.	www.cqvip
ClinicalTrials.gov	—	Clinical trial registry.	https://clinicaltrials.gov
Cochrane Central Register of Controlled Trials	CENTRAL	Bibliographic database that provides a highly concentrated source of reports of randomised controlled trials.	http://community.cochrane.org/ editorial-and-publishing-policy-resource/cochrane-central-register-controlled-trials-central
Combination therapies	—	Two or more Chinese medicines from different therapy groups (Chinese herbal medicine, acupuncture therapies or other Chinese medicine therapies) administered together.	—
Convention on International Trade in Endangered Species of Wild Fauna and Flora	CITES	—	www.cites.org/eng/disc/text.php
Cumulative Index of Nursing and Allied Health Literature	CINAHL	Bibliographic database.	www.ebscohost.com/nursing/about

(*Continued*)

Glossary of Terms	Abbreviation	Definition	Reference
Effect size	—	A generic term for the estimate of effect of treatment for a study.	http://handbook.cochrane.org
Episodic migraine	—	Episodic migraine occurs on less than 15 days per month and can be further subdivided into low frequency (1–9 days per month) and high frequency (10–14 days per month).	Headache Classification Committee of the International Headache Society (IHS). (2013) The International Classification of Headache Disorders, 3rd ed. (beta version). *Cephalalgia* **33(9):** 629–808.
Excerpta Medica dataBASE	Embase	Bibliographic database.	www.elsevier.com/solutions/embase
Grading of Recommendations Assessment, Development, and Evaluation	GRADE	Approach to grading certainty (quality) of evidence and strength of recommendations.	www.gradeworkinggroup.org
Headache Impact Test–6	HIT–6	A brief tool for assessing the impact of headache in both clinical research and practice.	Rendas-Baum R, Yang M, Varon SF, *et al.* (2014) Validation of the Headache Impact Test (HIT–6) in patients with chronic migraine. *Health Qual Life Outcomes* **1(12):** 117.
Heterogeneity	—	Used in a general sense to describe the variation in, or diversity of, participants, interventions and measurement of outcomes across a set of studies, or the variation in internal validity of those studies. Used specifically, as statistical heterogeneity, to describe the degree of variation in the effect estimates from a set of studies. Also used to indicate the presence of variability among studies beyond the amount expected due solely to chance.	http://handbook.cochrane.org

(*Continued*)

(Continued)

Glossary of Terms	Abbreviation	Definition	Reference
I^2	—	A measure of study heterogeneity, indicating the percentage of variance in a meta-analysis.	http://handbook.cochrane.org
Mean difference	MD	In meta-analysis, a method used to combine measures on continuous scales, where the mean, standard deviation and sample size in each group are known. The weight given to the difference in means from each study (e.g. how much influence each study has on the overall results of the meta-analysis) is determined by the precision of its estimate of effect; mathematically this is equal to the inverse of the variance. This method assumes that all of the trials have measured the outcome on the same scale.	http://handbook.cochrane.org
Meta-analysis	—	The use of statistical techniques in a systematic review to integrate the results of included studies. Sometimes misused as a synonym for a systematic review, where the review includes a meta-analysis.	—
Migraine Disability Assessment	MIDAS	A questionnaire to determine how severely migraines affect patients' quality of life.	Stewart WF, Lipton RB, Dowson AJ, *et al.* (2001) Development and testing of the Migraine Disability Assessment (MIDAS) Questionnaire to assess headache-related disability. *Neurology* **56(6 Suppl 1):** S20–S28.

(Continued)

Glossary of Terms	Abbreviation	Definition	Reference
Migraine-Specific Quality-of-Life Questionnaire	MSQ	A questionnaire containing 14 items to assess the effects of migraine and its treatment on patients' health-related quality of life.	Jhingran P, Davis SM, LaVange LM, *et al.* (1998) MSQ: Migraine-Specific Quality-of-Life Questionnaire. Further investigation of the factor structure. *Pharmacoeconomics.* **13**(6):707–717.
Moxibustion	—	A therapeutic procedure involving ignited material (usually *moxa*) to apply heat to certain points or areas of the body surface for curing disease through regulation of the function of meridians/channels and visceral organs.	World Health Organisation. (2007) WHO International Standard Terminologies of Traditional Medicine in the Western Pacific Region.
Non-randomised controlled clinical trial	CCT	An experimental study in which people are allocated to different interventions using methods that are not random.	http://handbook.cochrane.org
Numeric rating scales	NRS	A subjective measure in which individuals rate their pain on an eleven-point numerical scale. The scale is composed of 0 (no pain at all) to 10 (worst imaginable pain).	Kjaer P, Kongsted A, Hartvigsen J, *et al.* (2017) National clinical guidelines for non-surgical treatment of patients with recent onset neck pain or cervical radiculopathy. *Eur Spine J* **26(9):** 2242–2257.
Other Chinese medicine therapies	—	Other Chinese medicine therapies including all traditional therapies except Chinese herbal medicine and acupuncture, such as *taichi* 太极, *qigong* 气功, Chinese pulmonary rehabilitation, *tuina* 推拿 and cupping.	—
PubMed	PubMed	Bibliographic database.	www.ncbi.nlm.nih.gov/pubmed

(Continued)

(*Continued*)

Glossary of Terms	Abbreviation	Definition	Reference
Randomised controlled trial	RCT	A study in which a number of similar people are randomly assigned to two (or more) groups to test a specific drug, treatment or other intervention. One group (the experimental group) has the intervention being tested, the other (the comparison or control group) has an alternative intervention, a dummy intervention (placebo) or no intervention at all. The groups are followed up to see how effective the experimental intervention was. Outcomes are measured at specific times and any difference in response between the groups is assessed statistically. This method is also used to reduce bias.	www.nice.org.uk/glossary
Risk of bias	—	Assessment of clinical trials to indicate whether the results may overestimate or underestimate the true effect because of bias in the study design or reporting.	http://handbook.cochrane.org
Risk ratio	RR	The ratio of risks in two groups. In intervention studies, it is the ratio of the risk in the intervention group to the risk in the control group. A risk ratio of 1 indicates no difference between comparison groups. For undesirable outcomes, a risk ratio that is less than 1 indicates the intervention was effective in reducing the risk of that outcome.	http://handbook.cochrane.org

Glossary

(*Continued*)

Glossary of Terms	Abbreviation	Definition	Reference
Scalp acupuncture	—	Acupuncture at the specific lines located on the scalp.	World Health Organisation. (2007) WHO International Standard Terminologies of Traditional Medicine in the Western Pacific Region.
Standardised mean difference	SMD	In meta-analysis, a method used to combine results for continuous scales which measure the same outcome, but in different ways (e.g. with different scales). The results of studies are standardised to a uniform scale to allow data to be combined.	http://handbook.cochrane.org
Summary of findings	SoF	Presentation of results and ratings of the quality of evidence based on the GRADE approach.	http://www.gradeworkinggroup.org
Tuina 推拿 therapy	—	Branch of traditional Chinese medicine concerned with the principles and clinical use of *tuina* (massage) therapy.	World Health Organisation. (2007) WHO International Standard Terminologies of Traditional Medicine in the Western Pacific Region.
Visual Analogue Scale	VAS	A continuous measurement instrument for subjective characteristics or attitudes that cannot be directly measured, such as pain intensity.	Flynn D, Schaik VP, Wersch AV. (2004) A comparison of multi-item Likert and visual analogue scales for the assessment of transactionally defined coping function. *Eur J Psychol Assess* **20(1):** 49–58.
Wanfang database	Wanfang	Chinese language bibliographic database.	www.wanfangdata.com
World Health Organisation	WHO	WHO is the directing and coordinating authority for health within the United Nations system. It is responsible for providing leadership on global health matters, shaping the health research agenda, setting norms and standards, articulating	http://www.who.int/about/en

(*Continued*)

(*Continued*)

Glossary of Terms	Abbreviation	Definition	Reference
		evidence-based policy options, providing technical support to countries and monitoring and assessing health trends.	
Zhong Hua Yi Dian 中华医典	ZHYD	The *Zhong Hua Yi Dian* [*Encyclopaedia of Traditional Chinese Medicine*] is a comprehensive series of electronic books on compact disk. It is the largest collection of Chinese electronic books and includes the major Chinese classical works, many of which are from rare manuscripts and are the only existing copies. These books cover the period from before the Tang dynasty to the period of the Republic of China (1911–1948).	Hu R, ed. (2014) *Zhong Hua Yi Dian* [*Encyclopaedia of Traditional Chinese Medicine*], 5th ed. Hunan Electronic and Audio-Visual Publishing House, Chengsha.
Zhong Yi Fang Ji Da Ci Dian 中医方剂大辞典	ZYFJDCD	Compendium of Chinese herbal formulas with over 96,592 entries derived from classical Chinese books. The Nanjing Chinese Medicine Institute compiled this and first published it in 1993.	Peng HR, ed. (1994) *Zhong Yi Fang Ji Da Ci Dian* [*Great Compendium of Chinese Medical Formulae*]. People's Medical Publishing House, Beijing.

Index

www.ingramcontent.com/pod-product-compliance
Ingram Content Group UK Ltd.
Pitfield, Milton Keynes, MK11 3LW, UK
UKHW021824150726
7214IPUK00017B/300